# Group Work
# with the Poor and Oppressed

The *Social Work with Groups* series

# Group Work
# with the Poor
# and Oppressed

Judith A. B. Lee
Editor

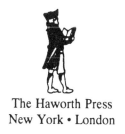

The Haworth Press
New York • London

*Group Work with the Poor and Oppressed* has also been published as *Social Work with Groups*, Volume 11, Number 4 1988.

The Haworth Press, Inc., 12 West 32 Street, New York, NY 10001
EUROSPAN/Haworth, 3 Henrietta Street, London WC2E 8LU England

**Library of Congress Cataloging-in-Publication Data**

Group work with the poor and oppressed.

"Has also been published as Social work with groups, volume 11, number 4, 1988" — T.p. verso.
Includes bibliographies.
1. Social group work — United States. 2. Social work with the homeless — United States. 3. Psychiatric social work — United States. 4. Social work with women — United States. I. Lee, Judith A. B.
HV45.G7318 1988    362.5'4'0973    88-32009
ISBN 0-86656-884-0

# Group Work
# with the Poor and Oppressed

## CONTENTS

**BOOK REVIEWS**

# ABOUT THE EDITOR

**Judith A. B. Lee, DWS,** currently Professor of Social Work at the University of Connecticut School of Social Work, has also taught at Columbia University and New York University. In addition to her role as educator, Dr. Lee has many years of experience as a social work practitioner. Most of her practice experience has been with poor and oppressed groups, including foster children, and the elderly and homeless women in the shelters of New York City. A recurring theme throughout her work is the creation and recreation of primary group ties as a healing force and as a vehicle for social action and social change. Dr. Lee is President of the Association for the Advancement of Social Work With Groups.

# Group Work
# with the Poor and Oppressed

# Preface

In its largest sense, this is a book about oppression and what social workers who work with groups of the vulnerable know and feel and do about powerlessness. More specifically, it is about the poor and the homeless and what those social workers know and feel and do about empowerment. For readers the book will yield increased knowledge of empowerment theory and practice (knowing) that can be generalized to work with all groups (doing), and increased understanding of the depth and extent of the contemporary social work commitment (feeling).

Judith A. B. Lee edited well: In contrast to many edited volumes, these authors manifest an unusual degree of thematic coherence centered on the professional objective of empowerment, while they present a rich diversity of practice skills that empower. Another source of unity lies in program development. For example, the practitioners are located in the life space of those being served: the SRO, shelter, soup kitchen, walk-in center, school, and the streets. And, finally, these social workers are not afraid to illustrate failure or error along with the successes.

Practice illustrations exemplify the structural approach of Middleman and Goldberg: Through group processes of mutual aid members are empowered by rediscovering and exercising their capacities for relatedness, competence, self-esteem, and self-direction to the degree possible. Some aspects of some of the harsh environments are humanized, and members' access to needed knowledge and skills is facilitated. Innovative life-space services are developed and funding secured. Implicit is the required participation of all social workers in social and policy change efforts so that the forces creating disempowerment, poverty, and homelessness are reduced.

*1*

Seasoned practitioners, social work students and educators will find this book fresh and exciting—as well as inspiring in its reflection of the heritage that pervades the distinguishing features of social work practice.

*Carel B. Germain, DSW*
*Emerita Professor of Social Work*
*University of Connecticut School of Social Work*

# Foreword

Judith A. B. Lee, "returned to the roots" of social group work well before the many of us, even those of us who have been outraged by the profession's seeming abandonment of the most wretched of our citizenry. Several years ago Lee put aside time from her busy academic schedule to use her proven group work skills with homeless women in the shelters of New York City (1983). She also undertook to reawaken in all of us our indebtedness to Jane Addams in the heritage of group work, indeed in the heritage of the social work profession (1987).

Judy Lee has gathered together practitioners and educators who possess a similar fervor and commitment to the forgotten multitude of our fellow humans who struggle to stay alive in the midst of the affluence of a society gone mad with abundance. These authors are younger social workers. They are not those of us whose professional group work lives were honed in the heyday of the settlements and Jewish Center movements. Rather they are social group workers who have developed their skills in the methodological era of the past three decades.

We offer this special collection to readers with pride. We also call the attention of our readers to the significant efforts of the Bertha Capen Reynolds Society to mobilize concerned persons in our profession into "a critical radical practice movement." By the time that this special collection on *Group Work with the Poor and Oppressed* is in the hands of readers there will have been held a second annual meeting of the BCR Society. Many groupworkers, treasuring Reynolds' belief in empowerment as an integral part of the helping profession, have participated in the sponsorship and growth of that organization.

As fellow editors we see this special collection, which Judy Lee has so ably edited, as testimony to empowerment as significant therapeutic experience and an essential value-based goal of the profession of social work. We highlight the statement by Enid Cox in her article conceptualizing the role of group work with the elderly poor, "Empowerment can not be achieved in isolation."

This collection presents historical, conceptual and practice content for group workers. It is also a contribution to all social workers whose ideological commitment is the maintenance of the profession's closeness to those most in need. It offers ideas and practice examples to stimulate the activity of our colleagues. It launches social work literature anew toward the exchange of creative experience in meeting human needs through the skills for working with the small group. It serves as an invitation to our colleagues to affirm the social group work tradition.

*Catherine P. Papell*
*Beulah Rothman*
*Editors*, Social Work with Groups

## NOTES

Lee, Judith A. B. "Who's Looking Out For The Homeless?" *NASW News* 28, No. 8 (September 1983): 4-5.

_____. "Social Work With Oppressed Populations: Jane Addams Won't You Please Come Home?" *Social Group Work: Competence and Values in Practice*. Joseph Lassner, Kathleen Powell, and Elaine Finnegan, Eds. New York: The Haworth Press, Inc., 1987, 1-16.

# Introduction:
# Return to Our Roots

Judith A. B. Lee

This collection is devoted to group work with the poor and oppressed. Whether we speak of the underclass (the term in Jane Addams' day was "the submerged tenth"), the welfare poor, the
working poor, the near poor or the new poor, we are clear that the
poor are oppressed and that group work is critical to empowering
them. Recent U.S. Census Bureau figures (1986) indicate that four
million adults receive welfare while 7 million are the working poor
(USN and WR, 1988). This does not account for children and youth
on welfare or for those who hover precariously just above the "poverty line" (always a pitifully low figure) such as the elderly living
on fixed incomes mentioned in Cox's astute article in this volume.
It does not account for the feminization of poverty noted by Breton
or the rate of unemployment in the black community noted by both
Cox and Parsons. It also does not account for those who subsist
without welfare as many of the nation's homeless do as described
by Martin and Nayowith, Berman-Rossi and Cohen in this volume.
Another recent statistic estimated 32 million poor in this country
(*Hartford Courant*, 1988). Figures on homelessness range from
Mitch Snyder's 3 million to *Fortune* magazine's victim blaming
article citing "not more than 500,000" (1987) as if the numbers
bear the weight of our inhumanity to our fellows. The point is societal and structural inhumanity and the response of social group
work to this oppression and to the double and triple oppressions of
gender, race, age, and illness (mental or physical) combined with
poverty.

Judith A. B. Lee, DSW, is Professor of Social Work, University of Connecticut School of Social Work.

5

The roots of social group work with the poor in the USA can be traced to the settlement movement, Jane Addams and the start of Hull House in 1889 as Pottick points out in her scholarly treatise in this volume. Addams was an intellectual activist and a sensitive humanist whose understanding of the reciprocal nature of human relationships, especially between classes, was well ahead of her times. According to Pottick, if we look at Hull House carefully, we can see group work in soup kitchens, a shelter for homeless, and abused women as well as the various clubs noted by Parsons, Glasser and Suroviak and Martin and Nayowith also in this volume. Addams' belief in "the solidarity of the human race" no matter who represents it (Addams, 1910, 1961) led her to living with the poor and the kind of acts of love (commitment) basic to work with the oppressed (Friere, 1973, 34).

> The oppressor is in solidary with the oppressed only when he stops regarding the oppressed as an abstract category and sees them as persons who have been unjustly dealt with, deprived of their voice, cheated in the sale of their labor—when he stops making pious . . . gestures and risks an act of love. (1973:34)

The oppressed poor are not to be seen as marginals

> . . . living outside society. They have always been inside—inside the structure which made them beings for others. The solution is not to integrate them into the structure of oppression but to transform the structure so they can become beings for themselves. (1973:61)

By Friere's definition, Jane Addams was a radical, one "not afraid to confront, to listen, to see the world unveiled . . . not afraid to meet the people or enter into dialogue with them . . . (the radical) does not consider himself . . . the liberator of the oppressed; but he does commit himself, within history, to fight at their side" (1973:24).

This side by sideness is a social group work position taken by Addams, and by each author represented in this volume. In Addams' method of neighboring and discussion (1932), Friere's *Peda-*

*gogy*, William Schwartz's belief in mutual aid (1974), Germain and Gitterman's life model approach (1980), and Papell and Rothman's mainstream model of group work (1978) there is a trust in people and their processes which argues a strikingly similar basis for social work practice with groups.

> Every human being is capable of looking critically at his world in dialogical encounters with others. . . . In this process, the old, paternalistic teacher-student (read worker-client/group member) relationship is overcome. . . . Each man wins back his own right to say his own word, to name the world. (Friere, 1973:13)

Further, "No one can say a true word alone – nor can he say it for another in a prescriptive act which robs others of their words. . . . Dialogue cannot be reduced to the act of one person's 'depositing' ideas in another, nor can it become a simple exchange of ideas . . ." (1973:76-77). As William Schwartz would often note, it is hard work.

Cox's thoughtful application of empowerment theory to groups of the elderly and Berman-Rossi and Cohen's careful documentation and critique of five years of group work with a dinner group of mentally ill women in an S.R.O. Hotel clearly show the struggle in both theory and practice to enable the group member to "say her own word." The old issue of "whose group is it?" is clear in group work with the oppressed. It cannot be the worker's for that is oppressive. It ultimately is the members', and in the process, belongs to both the worker and the members in equal dialogue with each other. Breton's struggle with the norms of a nurturing agency and its reluctance to encourage groups to form and develop is still another honest attempt at moving away from a charity model and "the banking notion" of helping (to deposit wisdom in others) which Friere considers contradictory to real dialogue, mutual aid, freedom and self-determination. The authors in this volume clearly agree with Breton's definition of mutual aid not as an end in itself but as an "empowering mechanism" relevant to political and personal change simultaneously. Parsons, Cox and Breton also use Friere's concept of consciousness raising as a critical part of their group work with three very different oppressed groups. Structured groups are also used creatively (Parsons, Cox, and Glasser and Suroviak) as a means of empowerment.

The concept of group work to promote social networks essential for survival and empowerment is beautifully explored and illustrated by Martin and Nayowith in a range of settings, from street work to working in a residential hotel, and by Glasser and Suroviak in the soup kitchen. The use of activities, or doing with, is noted by all of the authors as a medium of work with group members. Empowering activities range from ethnic food celebrations, trips, leadership development classes, bingo, cooking and dinner groups to confronting authoritative agencies and attending social protests (see Middleman, 1983). The operative word here, as dramatically pointed out in Berman-Rossi and Cohen's article and Friere's classical work is doing *with*, since the process itself, including the worker's every action must be empowering, not just the hoped for outcomes.

A strong solid research component is built into Parson's article which demonstrates well that the empowering effects of mutual aid groups can be measured and positive findings obtained. A rigorous evaluative look at programs over time is demonstrated in all of the articles.

In short, this is a very special volume which promises the reader a front-line view of social group work with the poor/oppressed. Its attempts to integrate our history and the present time, and empowerment, liberation, and radical social work theories, ecological and anthropological approaches, and basic social group work theory with practice with a variety of groups ranging from minority teenage girls, to homeless women and men, in and out of hotels, and guests in soup kitchens, and the elderly make it a volume of unusual depth and breadth. It does not pretend to offer examples of ideal practice, for the state of the art in integrating this range of theory with social group work practice with the oppressed poor does not yet permit this. We are learning, we are trying, and we are side by side once again with the poor. If nothing else, this volume says we have reclaimed our roots and are where we need to be.

# REFERENCES

Addams, J., *Twenty Years At Hull House*, New York: A Signet Classic, 1961, p. 98 (1910).

*Fortune Magazine*, "Homeless," M. Magnet, November 23, 1987, pp. 170-190.

Friere, P., *Pedagogy of the Oppressed*, New York: The Seabury Press, 1973.

Germain, Carel B. and Gitterman, Alex. *The Life Model of Social Work Practice*, New York: Columbia, 1980.

*Hartford Courant*, March 19, 1988, "God Bless the Child . . . "

Middleman, R., Ed., "Activities and Action In Group Work," *Social Work With Groups*, Vol. 6(1) Spring, 1983.

Papell, C., and Rothman, B. "Relating the Mainstream Model of Social Work with Groups to Group Psychotherapy and the Structured Group Approach," *Social Work with Groups*, Vol. 3(2) Summer, 1980: 5-22.

Schwartz, W., "The Social Worker In The Group," in W. Klenk and W. Ryan, Eds. *The Practice of Social Work*, Belmont Calif.: Wadsworth, 1974, pp. 208, 228.

*U.S. News and World Report*, "America's Hidden Poor," Jan. 11, 1988, pp. 18-24.

# Jane Addams Revisited:
# Practice Theory and Social Economics

## Kathleen J. Pottick

**SUMMARY.** This paper presents Jane Addams' challenge to commonly held assumptions promoted by the industrialists of the 1890s about the means to secure democracy and national progress. The paper focuses on her alternate conception and her practice model deriving from this conception. The historical analysis provides a framework to view leadership for contemporary theory building.

This paper is not about groups. It is not about group functioning, group development or group practice. It is about the practice of a social worker to whom most group workers owe their legacy and heritage. It is about Jane Addams. On a particular level, the paper focuses on how the social thought of her times influenced her to think about certain social problems and how she came to develop her practice in response to the social thought of the times. It details her innovative attack on the assumptions of the 1890s accepted philanthropic thinking advocated by a generation of "Big Businessmen" and describes how she came to view the contemporary social thought as a social problem itself. On a general level, the paper suggests that leadership in social work, such as that demonstrated by Jane Addams, develops out of the ability to conceptualize contemporary social thought and to create practice ideas articulated in that context.

Jane Addams' model of social work is presented here as an illus-

Kathleen J. Pottick is affiliated with Rutgers University School of Social Work, 536 George Street, New Brunswick, NJ 08903.

The author would like to thank Miriam Dinerman, Harold Demone, Ludwig Geismar, Judy Lee and Rush Welter for their comments and suggestions on an earlier version of the text.

tration of a model which embraced major social goals, but challenged the accepted means to secure those goals. Perhaps it is for this reason that Jane Addams and other reform-minded historical leaders have captured the attention of contemporary social work thinkers. For example, Axinn (1983) focuses on two reform periods — the Progressive era in the early twentieth century and the 1960s — to understand the conditions under which reform takes place. More recently, at the ninth symposium of the Association for the Advancement of Social Work with Groups, Lee (1987) forwards Jane Addams' ideas about practice as approaches worth considering and applying today. As social workers come to understand and struggle to ameliorate social problems on a scale unimaginable at the turn of the last century, they also can draw inspiration and strength from exceptional historical figures. Jane Addams is one such figure. Moreover, while the identification of important historical moments in the development of social work is interesting in its own right, it may also serve to help us create and adopt new social work knowledge.

## JANE ADDAMS' FIRST THIRTY YEARS

By 1900 Jane Addams had gained a national reputation among the major political and social theorists of the time. Ten years earlier, she established Hull House, one of the first settlement houses in the United States. She was twenty-nine at the time, by today's standards a young person.

She was born into a family of some means, the daughter of an Illinois miller, John Addams. She was the youngest of eight children. Her mother, Sarah, died before Jane was three years old, and her father remarried when Jane was eight. According to Jane Addams' nephew, her most authoritative biographer, she was "small, frail, and pigeon-toed, and carried her head slightly on one side as the result of a slight spinal curvature" (Linn, 1935, p. 24). She was chronically ill throughout her life, and underwent several operations on her spine and intestines.

Jane Addams attended Rockford Seminary (later Rockford College). Although she was encouraged to enter a career in missionary work, she decided instead to study medicine at the Women's Medical College in Philadelphia. She did not complete her studies, ill-health forcing her to withdraw.

Jane Addams' father died in her last year at the seminary. According to her biographers, her father's death affected her very deeply. With her father's death and her medical problems, she sank into a depression, not to fully recover until she founded Hull House seven years after she left the medical college (Linn, 1935; Tims, 1961). During those seven years she visited Europe twice — the first trip with her stepmother, the second trip alone. It was during this second trip that she came to develop the idea of creating a settlement house in the United States, much in the fashion of Toynbee Hall — the London settlement she visited. Over the seven years, Jane Addams became increasingly despondent — she attempted to search out culture only to discover further loneliness and isolation. Reflecting on the time she left Rockford in 1881 until she went to Hull House in 1889, Jane Addams said that she was "absolutely at sea so far as any moral purpose was concerned, clinging only to the desire to live in a really living world and refusing to be content with a shadowy intellectual or esthetic reflection of it" (Linn, 1935, p. 65). Jane Addams' essay, "The Subjective Necessity for Social Settlements" from her book *Philanthropy and Social Progress* (1893), describes her feeling that pursuing culture for its own sake is a futile effort that had driven women like herself into the settlement movement (Lasch, 1965).

## *LIFE AT HULL HOUSE*

Jane Addams spent five months looking for a building to begin her "project" as she referred to it. She finally found a house — on Halsted Street — a "big house down among the little houses" (Linn, 1935, p. 91). It had been built as a suburban residence in 1856 by Charles J. Hull when Chicago's population was 85,000. The house was brick, two-storied, with a great front entrance, large rooms, high ceiling, mahogany throughout, and a piazza that circled the house. The house originally stood in countryside, but by the time Jane Addams rented it, the population was nearly one million, the second largest city (New York was the first) in the United States. When Jane Addams and Ellen Gates Starr and a housekeeper, Mary

Keyser, moved into the house on September 14, 1889, over 700,000 people in Chicago were foreign-born. In the 1890 census, only 292,000 Americans were listed, including 15,000 blacks. There were 215,000 Irish and 400,000 Germans. Twenty thousand Italians were listed, and about ten thousand Italians and thousands upon thousands of Irish were said to live in the area surrounding Hull House (Linn, 1935, pp. 91-96).

Jane Addams' description of the neighborhood of the house and the surrounding area reveals her interests, her observational skills, and the problems she endeavored to solve:

> Halsted Street is thirty-two miles long. . . . Polk Street crosses it midway between the stockyards to the south and the ship-building yards on the north branch of the Chicago river. For the six miles between these industries the street is lined with shops of butchers and grocers, with dingy and gorgeous saloons, and pretentious establishments for the sale of ready-made clothing. Polk Street, west from Halsted, grows rapidly more prosperous; running a mile east to State Street it grows steadily worse, and crosses a network of vice on the corners of Clark Street and Fifth Avenue. . . . The streets are inexpressibly dirty, the number of schools inadequate, sanitary legislation unenforced, the street lighting bad, the paving miserable and altogether lacking in the alleys and smaller streets, and the stables foul beyond description. Hundreds of houses are unconnected with the street sewer. . . . The houses, for the most part wooden, were originally built for one family and are now occupied by several. They are after the type of the inconvenient frame cottages found in the poorer suburbs before the Fire. Many of them were built where they now stand; others were brought there on rollers, because their previous sites had been taken for factories . . . .The little wooden houses have a temporary aspect, and for this reason, perhaps, the tenement-house legislation in Chicago is totally inadequate. Rear tenements flourish; many houses have no water supply save the faucet in the back yard, there are no fire escapes, the garbage and ashes are placed in wooden boxes which are fastened to the street pavements. (Linn, 1935, p. 97)

Jane Addams lacked money for her project, and she relied on donations and payment for public speaking engagements — "talks" as she called them (Linn, 1935, p. 104). She impressed many with her earliest efforts to establish a neighborhood center. In 1890, just one year after the project started, Helen Culver, the cousin and sole heir to the four million dollar estate of Charles J. Hull, granted Jane Addams a free five-year lease.

The first year proved to be an important one. In that first year, over 50,000 people made use of the house. In the second year, an average of 2,000 people visited Hull House weekly. Within five years of its creation, Hull House had a staff of fifteen resident workers. In addition to Ellen Gates Starr, the distinguished group of early workers included Julia Lathrop, Florence Kelly, and Alice Hamilton (Tims, 1961, pp. 55-56).

Hull House activities included reading groups (children during the day, adults in the evening), arts and crafts classes, Sunday concerts, and a women's labor club. (Called the "Jane Club," this club developed into a cooperative boarding club for working girls.) A public kitchen was established to provide cheap and nutritious meals for housewives and workers. In addition, a coffee house and a children's playground were created and a nursery and kindergarten (to accommodate working mothers) were developed.

It was in the context of the influx of immigrants to Chicago that Jane Addams' project was initiated. She was concerned about the consequences of immigration — the sociological and psychological effects of relocation — on individuals and families. She was concerned with helping foreign-born people establish an American identity, and she was concerned with helping foreign-born people pass on their unique heritage to their children. Maintaining individuals' ethnic roots and enriching the ever-changing heritage of America were goals that she strived to attain through the activities at Hull House.

While immigration was on the rise in the late 1800s, so too was social invention, and an increasing division of rich and poor. Most of Chicago's wealth was centered in the hands of the thirty percent of the American born — the meat packers: the Armours, Swifts, and Libbys; or the merchants: the Bartletts, Cranes, Fairbanks, Fields, Kimballs, Pullmans, Rosenwalds, and Wentworths, to name a few — and they were the power brokers in Chicago (Linn, 1935, p. 100).

The tension between business and the labor became pronounced. Labor unions were "fought on principle," and some of the more outspoken came to be marked as "anarchists" for conspiracy. As Linn (1935) puts it, "In 1889 Chicago was eminently class-conscious and blood-conscious. It was a house divided. The small governing American minority was profoundly suspicious of the vast governed immigrant majority" (p. 102). Yet, this small minority was an influential group, a group that had a well-articulated view of the requisites for the creation and maintenance of wealth, national progress, and American success.

It was in this broad social context that Jane Addams began her activities at Hull House, her public speaking, and her own writing.

## JANE ADDAMS AS INTELLECTUAL ACTIVIST

Jane Addams' first book, *Democracy and Social Ethics*, published in 1902, marked her as an intellectual. That book represents an inquiry into the cultures of the working and middle classes and describes how misconceptions between the classes are maintained. It also details the problems in the "helping relation," — inevitable problems between people attempting to understand each others' motives for either giving help or receiving it. She thought that all behavior could be understood if the goal or value or motive of the individual were understood. Such a view allowed her to align herself with both classes because she was able to describe what it was that each class or individual in a class was attempting to obtain. (In contemporary terms, we might say that she was expressing an early conceptualization of the mediating function in social work.) The book outlines her criticisms of the efforts of the "friendly visitors," a criticism aimed directly at the methods of local charity. The historian Christopher Lasch (1965) says that her book "struck some of her contemporaries with the force of a revelation" (p. 62). It is difficult to believe that such an outcome was unintended. Her decisions about her life seem somehow deliberate.

She wrote nine books in her lifetime — *Democracy and Social Ethics* (1902), *Newer Ideals of Peace* (1907), *Twenty Years at Hull*

*House* (1910), *A New Conscience and an Ancient Evil* (1912), *The Long Road of Woman's Memory* (1916), *Peace and Bread in Time of War* (1922), *Second Twenty Years at Hull House* (1930), *The Excellent Becomes the Permanent* (1932) and *My Friend, Julia Lathrop* (1935). She also wrote scores of articles and speeches. Her books reflect the development of her thinking and her unfolding interests. In the early part of the twentieth century she became involved in the Progressive Movement and became an ardent supporter of pacifism during World War I. She is probably better remembered for her peace activities (she visited heads of state abroad during the war to promote peace) than for her earlier activities at Hull House. But it is about her earlier activities that this paper is concerned. For it was in those early papers and books that her intellectual struggle about working with people is articulated. Her books demonstrate how her activities are grounded in her thinking; her practice demonstrates how her thinking is grounded in her activities. All of her books, including the last one, a biography of her good friend, Julia Lathrop, appear to be inspired by a desire to express herself in writing. Her sensitive practice and her thoughtful writing about her practice seem somehow linked. Her essays and books develop a new way to understand social relations; and it seems that she hoped that by influencing people to think differently that they might act differently. In fact, in *Peace and Bread in Time of War*, she says that "the activities of life can be changed in no other way than by changing the current ideas upon which it is conducted" (p. 243).

## THE TENOR OF THE 1890s

The late nineteenth century of American history witnessed the emergence of the "captains of industry" — such men as Andrew Carnegie, Commodore Cornelius Vanderbilt, Jay Gould, and George Pullman, the founders of capitalist fortunes and the first American business heroes. To many Americans, these self-made men became mythical hero images. To pore over the pages of speeches written by these men is to view a powerful declaration of their ideas about the relationship between individual success, national progress and democracy. The accumulation of fortunes by a few worthy, exceptional, and moral individuals and by the growth of consolidated industry under their auspices was the foundation of the "gospel of wealth."

According to the big businessmen, democracy was demonstrated by the ability of individuals to rise out of their circumstances, however humble they might have been. Carl Sandburg (1886) expressed this predominant belief in egalitarianism. He said that America was the "one country in the world where it (was) possible for a man to rise by his own effort from obscurity and poverty not only to the highest place in society, but also to the courted rank of millionaire as well." In contrast to an earlier era where "labor" was considered the key to the creation of wealth, in this era "the mind" was heralded as the real creator of wealth. Orville Platt (1881) makes this point clearly in his essay "Invention and Advancement":

> a brigade of workmen cannot do as much effective good as is done by one strong capitalist, whose money employs and whose sagacity directs and renders fruitful the sterile hand.

Considered essential to the national progress was the creation of wealth. By creating more businesses and more jobs through consolidated industry, the big businessmen reasoned they created more opportunities for personal, community and social advancement. For example, Andrew Carnegie (1889) proposed that the "masses of people are just as comfortable as the proportion of millionaires." It was Carnegie's belief, and that of most of the other industrialists, that amassed wealth would trickle down to the entire nation.

The industrialists' aim was to educate the masses through philanthropic giving. Philanthropic efforts supposedly ensured the education of the masses whose lack of culture constrained industriousness. Thus, the "big businessmen" established universities, libraries, museums, and trusts for the public good, activities that would serve to uplift the masses.

Philanthropic activities were seen as a natural outgrowth of the unequal distribution of wealth; and the unequal distribution of wealth was seen as a demonstration of national progress. For example, Andrew Carnegie (1889), pointing out the vast gap between the rich and poor, extolled the virtues of the existing social and economic structure for the benefit of civilization and progress of the race:

> The contrast between the palace of the millionaire and the cottage of the laborer with us today measures the change which has come with civilization. This change, however, is not to be deplored, but welcomed as highly beneficial. It is well, nay, essential for the progress of the race, that the houses of some should be homes for all that is highest and best in literature and the arts, and for all the refinements of civilization, rather than that none should be so. Much better this irregularity than universal squalor . . . The "Good Old Times" were not good old times. Neither master nor servant was as well situated then as today. A relapse to old conditions would be disastrous to both . . . not the least to him who serves — and would sweep away civilization with it.

Democracy was seen as a basic necessity for the progress of the race. The democratic system allowed the big businessman to rise from "humble" circumstances; it allowed him to provide for the rest of the masses. Providing to the masses through philanthropic efforts gave individuals an opportunity to rise themselves. When the masses as a group were elevated, and some individuals within that group able to rise, then progress would occur. Thus, democracy and national progress were thought to be secured and maintained by the outcomes of the distribution of wealth in the 1890s.

## AN ALTERNATE CONCEPTION

While the big businessmen hailed the unequal distribution of wealth and philanthropy as essential to the democratic process, Jane Addams was skeptical. In fact, Jane Addams began to view philanthropy as a potential social problem, dysfunctional to the attainment of democracy and national progress.

The Pullman Strike was one incident on which she could comment about relations between industrialists and laborers. Speaking of the rebellion which broke out in the town of Pullman by the railroad workers living in the model city, Jane Addams (1912) says:

The president of the Pullman company thought out within his own mind a beautiful town. He had power with which to build this town, but he did not appeal to nor obtain the consent of the men who were living in it. The most unambitious reform, recognizing the necessity for this consent, makes for slow but sane and strenuous progress, while the most ambitious of social plans and experiments, ignoring this, is prone to the failure of the model town of Pullman.

Philanthropy without the recognition of others' wants inhibited democracy because it limited the control and decision-making power individuals could have over their own lives. Thus, Jane Addams (1912) says that the town might well have worked if "he had called upon them (workmen) for self-expression and had made the town a growth and manifestation of their wants and needs." Jane Addams (1912) argued that philanthropy was a means by which control through giving could be exercised and that it had detrimental effects necessarily leading to failure. Calling Pullman "a modern Lear," Jane Addams says: ". . . so long as they (philanthropists) are 'good to people,' rather than 'with them' they are bound to accomplish a large amount of harm."

Local charity was another object of Jane Addams' concern. She thought that self-righteous control exercised from those people in more powerful positions in society could potentially stifle individuality and personal creativity. Speaking of the friendly visitors, Jane Addams (1902) remarked:

> But in our charitable efforts we think much more of what a man ought to be than of what he is or what he may become; and we ruthlessly force our conventions and standards upon him, with a sternness which we would consider stupid indeed did an educator use it in forcing his mature intellectual convictions.

Thus, the democratic standard of participatory freedom was undermined by decisional control exercised by those who forced their authority on recipients.

Philanthropic giving had far-reaching social repercussions, according to Jane Addams (1893). For one, it caused disharmonious social relations by expanding the social distance between the rich and the poor. To have the society so divided functioned to perpetuate the social problem, philanthropic giving.

> It is constantly said that because the masses have never had social advantages they do not want them . . . and that it will take political or philanthropic machinery to change them. This divides the city into rich and poor, into the favored, who express their sense of social obligation by gifts of money, and into the unfavored, who express it by clamoring for a "share" — both of them activated by a vague sense of justice.

Both givers and receivers, tenaciously holding distinct social roles and motivated by mutually destructive self-righteous indignation, undermined both personal growth and societal change, requisites of increased democratization and national progress.

Although Jane Addams did not reject capitalist giving as a means to foster social development (she accepted donations to support Hull House activities), she did reject philanthropic giving when it was given without regard to the wants of the recipient. In Jane Addams' view the dangers of philanthropy were threefold. First, philanthropic giving potentially limited recipients' ability to chart the course of their own lives, undermining self-determination and growth-producing decisional control. Second, philanthropic giving could undercut recipients' self-respect by undervaluing their potential contribution to and involvement with matters which affected their lives. Democratic life would suffer under these conditions. Third, philanthropic giving could contribute to social stagnation. Cut off from each others' experiences, both givers and receivers would retain unchangeable social positions. Since change is the prerequisite of progress, national growth and advancement would suffer at the hands of philanthropic giving.

## THE MODEL FOR PRACTICE

Jane Addams believed, as did the big businessmen, that individual creativity would promote national progress. But in her view, philanthropic giving was not the best means by which individual creativity would be attained. Rather, individual creativity was squelched by the outcomes of philanthropic giving — the undermining of self-determination and self-respect, as well as increased social stagnation. Giving based on reciprocity between the classes, an intimate interdependence which could be realized through education, was the means by which individual creativity could be promoted and democracy and national progress could flourish. In other words, the problems associated with philanthropic giving could be resolved if a model of giving based on a philosophy of reciprocity could be adopted. The test of the model was accomplished at Hull House. The philosophy of giving based on reciprocity was the operational basis of Hull House. According to Jane Addams (1893):

> Hull House endeavors to make social intercourse express the growing sense of the economic unity of society. It is an effort to add the social function to democracy. It was opened on the theory that the dependence of classes on each other is reciprocal.

It was the purpose of reciprocity to enlighten the social classes: "To shut oneself away from half the race life is to shut oneself away from the most vital part of it." In terms of learning and growth, the givers and receivers were interchangeable. Thus, middle-class friendly visitors working with lower-class individuals had much to learn from them regarding their culture. Differences in behavior and attitudes were viewed as understandable and logical outgrowths of cultural and economic variations within the social structure. This functional view of behavior was applied equally to all the social classes as a way of developing common understanding leading to greater recognition of the mutuality of experience. In one of her most powerful and sensitive pieces, Jane Addams (1902) addresses this issue:

> The subject of clothes indeed perplexes the friendly visitor constantly, and the result of her reflections may be summed up somewhat in this wise: "The girl who has a definite social standing, who has been to a fashionable school or to a college, . . . may afford to be very simple, or even shabby as to her clothes, if she likes. But the working girl, whose family lives

in a tenement, . . . knows full well how much habit and style of dress has to do with her position. Her income goes into her clothing out of all proportion to the amount which she spends on other things. But if social advancement is her aim, it is the most sensible thing she can do. . . ."

The charity visitor has been rightly brought up to consider it vulgar to spend much money on clothes, to care so much for 'appearance.' She realizes dimly that the care for personal decoration over that for one's own home or habitat is in some way primitive and undeveloped, but she is silenced by its obvious need.

A reciprocal exchange of learning which defined the nature of the relationship also had repercussions for the role of the worker and the nature of the tasks to be accomplished. In this model which Jane Addams (1893) describes the giver took the role of an enabler:

> . . . working people require only that their aspirations be recognized and stimulated, and the means of attaining them put at their disposal . . . Hull House . . . secure(s) these means for its neighbors, but to call that effort philanthropy is to use the word unfairly and to underestimate the duties of good citizenship.

The role of the worker was to provide an environment where individuals could engage themselves in decisions regarding their own lives. Self-determination was an integral part of the work; the giver did not dictate or control through giving the life wants and needs of the receiver.

According to Jane Addams (1893) the giver provided opportunities for the residents of Hull House to create their own program to serve their needs: "The residents of Hull House find in themselves a constantly increasing tendency to consult their neighbors on the adviseability of each new undertaking." At Hull House were available cultural days (e.g., German days, Italian days) where people from the neighborhood came to sing around the piano. As Jane Addams (1899) suggests, the social activities at Hull House were "an attempt to express the meaning of life in terms of life itself, in forms of activity." Educational, humanitarian, and civic programs, ranging from classes in English and geography to a community run day care program were initiated. The promoting of individual decision-making was seen as a way to develop more creative, free-thinking and independent individuals. Free-thinking, creative, independent people were those who could rise out of their circumstances. But since Jane Addams saw the acquisition of knowledge of other cultures as providing individual enhancement, receivers as well as the givers were the recipients of growth producing knowledge. The social stagnation reflected in immutable social roles of "giver" and "receiver" would be invariably reduced as reciprocal interdependence was fostered, nurtured, and maintained.

## CONCLUSION

Jane Addams' practice model represented a departure from the social thought of the era. In her view, philanthropic giving perpetuated social stagnation and undermined self-determination, thereby thwarting national progress and social democracy. Her model attempted to promote democracy and national progress by increasing individual self-determination and self-respect and decreasing social stagnation. By defining the proper nature of the giving relationship as reciprocal, rather than philanthropic, Jane Addams challenged commonly held assumptions about the means to secure democracy and national progress.

Any model of social work practice is distinguished by its own unique historical context. The goals it promotes and the means it fosters to attain the goals are developed in a social context. Jane Addams concurred with and embraced the goals of democracy and progress, but viewed the socially accepted way to secure these goals as a potential social problem itself. Viewing how models of practice develop in their social context may help us to understand the way social problems come to be addressed and solutions come to be proposed. It may also help us to question the nature of the social problems we seek to solve. And further, it may help us to ask whether dominant-culture solutions can suffice or whether social work will have to employ more innovative solutions.

# REFERENCES

*Primary Sources*

Addams, J. A modern Lear. *The Survey*, Vol. XXIX, November 2, 1912, pp. 131-137. In C. Lasch (Ed.), *The Social Thought of Jane Addams*, New York: The Bobbs-Merrill Company, Inc., 1965, pp. 105-123.

Addams, J. *Peace and Bread in Time of War*. New York: The Macmillan Company, 1932.

Addams, J. *Democracy and Social Ethics*, New York: The Macmillan Company, 1902, pp. 13-25, 30-41, 44-51, 58-70.

Addams, J. The subjective necessity for social settlements. *Philanthropy and Social Progress*. New York: Thomas Y. Crowell, Inc., 1893, pp. 1-26, In C. Lasch (Ed.), *The Social Thought of Jane Addams*, New York: The Bobbs-Merrill Company, Inc., 1965, pp. 28-43.

Addams, J. The objective value of a social settlement. *Philanthropy and Social Progress*, New York: Thomas Y. Crowell, Inc., 1893, pp. 27-40, In C. Lasch (Ed.), *The Social Thought of Jane Addams*, New York: The Bobbs-Merrill Company, Inc., 1965, pp. 44-61.

Addams, J. The function of a social settlement. *Annals of the American Academy of Political and Social Science*, Vol. XIII, May 1899, pp. 323-355, In C. Lasch (Ed.), *The Social Thought of Jane Addams*, New York: The Bobbs-Merrill Company, Inc., 1965, pp. 62-84.

Anonymous, A railroad eulogy. *New York Herald*, January 6, 1877, p. 3. In H.N. Smith (Ed.), *Popular Culture and Industrialism: 1865-1890*. New York: Doubleday & Company Inc., 1967, pp. 125-129.

Carnegie, A. A talk to young men, Address to the students of Curry Commercial College, Pittsburgh, June 23, 1885, In M. Curtis, W. Thorp, & C. Baker (Eds.), *American Issues: The Social Record*, 4th Ed. New York: J.P. Lippincott & Company, 1960, pp. 728-731.

Carnegie, A. Wealth. *North American Review*, June 1889, 148, pp. 91-100. In G. N. Grob & R. N. Beck (Eds.). *American Ideas: Source Readings in the Intellectual History of the United States. Vol. II (Dilemmas of maturity: 1865-1962)*. New York: The Free Press, pp. 91-100.

Gould, J. Testimony before the Senate committee on education and labor, New York, September 5, 1883. Report of the committee, Vol. I, pp. 1062-1068. In H.N. Smith (Ed.), *Popular Culture and Industrialism: 1865-1890*. New York: Doubleday & Company, Inc., 1967, pp. 130-139.

Platt, O.H. Invention and advancement. In Patent Centennial Celebration, Proceedings and addresses: Celebration of the beginning of the second century of the American patent system at Washington City, D.C., April 8,9,10, 1891. Washington, 1892, pp. 57-76. In H.N. Smith (Ed.), *Popular Culture and Industrialism: 1865-1890*, New York: Doubleday & Company, Inc., 1967, pp. 33-50.

*Collateral Sources*

Axinn, J. Women, social work and social reform, In M. Dinerman (Ed.) *Social Work Futures*. New Brunswick, NJ: Rutgers University Publications, 1983, pp. 79-95.

Lee, Judith A.B. Jane Addams in Boston: Intersecting Time and Space, Plenary speech, Ninth Symposium, Association for the Advancement of Social Work with Groups, Boston, MA, October 31, 1987.

Linn, James Weber. *Jane Addams*. New York: D. Appleton-Century Company, 1935.

Tims, Margaret. *Jane Addams of Hull-House*. London: George Allen & Unwin, 1961.

# Empowerment for Role Alternatives for Low Income Minority Girls: A Group Work Approach

Ruth J. Parsons

**SUMMARY.** This program was created to reach girls who may not believe they have control over their lives and are unfamiliar with alternative roles for women, making them high risk for adolescent pregnancy. An empowerment intervention framework was used to develop educational and mutual aid activities directed toward four major social systems identified as significant problem-solving areas for adolescents. In addition to program description, group processes such as composition, norms, cohesion and conflict resolution are discussed. Evaluation results are given.

## PROBLEM EXPLORATION

Adolescent pregnancy is a problem of significant proportions and of growing concern. While evaluation of attempts to affect the incidence of adolescent pregnancy has been inconclusive, Scales' (1979) review of programs to decrease adolescent pregnancy emphasized the need to recognize multiple causation of teen pregnancy and the importance of considering new and innovative models which address more than one causal factor. The Youth Values Project of the Population Institute of New York (Ross, 1979) reported that adolescent girls who are sexually active, but do not use birth control, can be categorized into three groups: (1) those who do not have contraceptive information; (2) those who have accurate information, but are not motivated to use it; and within that group, (3)

Ruth J. Parsons, PhD is Assistant Professor in the Graduate School of Social Work, University of Denver, University Park, Denver, CO 80208-0274.

those who choose to have a baby (or believe that is what the future holds) as a way of assuming the adult female role. This group was identified as a key to the high rate of pregnancy among economically disadvantaged minority girls (Simmons and Parsons, 1983). Lack of alternative role models, information, skills, and confidence to pursue alternatives to pregnancy as an entry to womanhood were thought to be barriers to girls' selection of alternative roles. Therefore, it was hypothesized that included in the multiple causal paradigm of adolescent pregnancy were two important empowerment concepts. One is an internal belief, locus of control, or internality, the belief or lack thereof that one has control over outcomes in one's life. This represents the internal attitude or psychological component of empowerment. The second aspect is knowledge and capacity to act in one's behalf to solve one's problems, an external component of empowerment. In a classist, sexist and racist society, low income minority girls find it difficult to believe they can be active participants in life's outcomes and they often lack access to resources.

The locus of control construct, developed by Rotter (1966), examined the degree to which people believe they have control over events in their lives. Internality represents the belief that one's own actions determine outcomes and consequences. Externality is the belief that situations and consequences are determined by luck, fate or powerful others. Work by Rotter concluded that poor people have less belief in control over their lives than non-poor; ethnic minorities perceive themselves to have less control than whites; and girls and women perceive themselves to have less control than men and boys. The major conclusions from studies regarding perception of control among children are that it increases with chronological age (Sherman, 1984), and that it is positively related to academic achievement in adolescents (Findley and Cooper, 1983). Other studies which compare adolescent attitudes and behavior with internality and externality orientations are inconclusive. Nowicki and Strickland (1973) found that fifth and sixth grade girls with higher internal locus of control also had higher achievement scores. Ross (1979) suggested that fatalistic attitudes toward pregnancy were related to lack of belief of control over life; however, Lieberman (1981) found that internality may not be of value in predicting contraceptive behavior. Robbins, Kaplan and Martin (1985) found no relationship between internality and adolescent pregnancy, and Young (1984) in a study of traditional, moderate and innovative career choices by girls, found no relationship to perception of control.

The question of whether perception of power and control over one's life is a variable in adolescent pregnancy is not resolved, yet the inclusion of the principle was still felt to be important. The problem exploration led to these programmatic goals: to broaden girls' horizons about women's roles; increase their knowledge and resources for women's role alternatives and increase their orientation to active problem solving on their own behalf. These were assumed to be critical, not only to the incidence of adolescent pregnancy, but also to girls' perception of themselves as women. Because values, beliefs, identity and self-assessment develop from association with others (Hartford, 1971), the small group was selected as the method of choice. Gitterman identified the enormous potential of mutual aid in the group as young people help each other negotiate the various systems with which they must come to terms (Gitterman, 1971). The purpose of the group was that of role attainment as a component of socialization. Groups organized for role attainment usually consist of members who seek similar socialization goals and are striving to overcome similar barriers to such achievement. Members are prone to identify strongly with, and give support to, one another in the process (Garvin, 1987).

Big Sisters, Inc., a private girls' agency whose programs are prevention oriented, created a small group program called Life Choices to achieve the goals stated above and intervened through the public schools with a six-month program. The intervention program was directed initially toward adolescent low-income minority girls. It was later expanded to a broader population of non-minorities and to various income levels as teen pregnancy goes across socioeconomic class and ethnic/racial lines.

## EMPOWERMENT: A THEORETICAL FRAMEWORK FOR INTERVENTION

The framework employed in the development of the program was based on Solomon's definition of empowerment (1976). She defined empowerment as the process of enabling persons to master their environment and achieve self-determination. Powerlessness, created by negative valuations based on membership in a stigmatized group, can be viewed as inability to manage skill, knowledge, and/or material resources in a way that effective performance of valued social roles will lead to personal gratification. The program was based on the assumption that low income minority girls are members of at least three stigmatized groups: women, ethnic, and poor. It was further assumed that they often lack knowledge, skill and confidence to access and manage resources in ways that enhance active problem solving and role attainment on their own behalf. Thus, it was assumed that the client group was disempowered in attitudes, real capacity and resources.

The concept of power in helping disadvantaged groups has been discussed widely in the literature. William Ryan (1972) perhaps best summarized the concept and its impact on individuals' perceptions of themselves. He suggested that power is a central component to self-esteem and survival of the human organism, and that a mentally healthy person must be able to perceive himself/herself as at least minimally powerful, capable of influencing his/her environment to his/her benefit, and that this sense of power had to be based upon the actual experience and exercise of power. Empowerment, while often measured as a psychological attitude of perceived confidence, and control, is both an internal and external process. The internal component is a psychological attitude, belief or feeling that one is competent to make decisions and solve one's own problems and dilemmas. The external component is the tangible knowledge, information, competences, skills and especially the resources which enable one to take action. The Life Choices program purpose was to decrease powerlessness, and increase perception of control by increasing girls' perceptions and beliefs about themselves as well as knowledge, skills, and resources for problem solving in their own lives. It was assumed that in order to increase girls' perceptions of power and ability to solve their own problems, the program would not only intervene at the attitudinal and belief level, but would also provide education about those most powerful social systems within which adolescent girls interact most frequently. Those were defined as: the health system, the vehicle of control of one's physical body;

peer relations; school system; and the beginning linkage to the economic system, career thinking and career choice. It was assumed that Ryan's concept of mastery of environment would most likely take place in those systems. Furthermore, it was assumed that education, awareness, knowledge and access to resources in these major systems were critical to empowerment of girls to become competent problem solvers on their own behalf.

## THE GROUP AS A SYSTEM OF MUTUAL AID

Selecting the small group as the method assumes that the clients have strengths to help and support each other to see themselves differently and learn skills through the mutual aid process to negotiate those more powerful systems.

William Schwartz proposed a general functional statement for the social work profession as that of mediating the social encounter. Small group is conceptualized as a microcosm of that encounter (Gitterman and Shulman, 1986). The social worker is the mediator of the mutual aid function both within the group and between the group and the larger systems which must be negotiated. Schwartz believed that society was made up of "complex ambivalent systems" that are hard to negotiate by all but the most skillful and best organized. He proposed that social work intervention appropriately provides a mediating or third force function (Lee, 1986) for people who need to attain resolution to their situations from those systems and who in turn must shape those systems and assist in their functioning. Life Choices provided girls with knowledge, skills and resources from those difficult to negotiate systems which impinge most upon their self-assessment and decision making behaviors. Thus, it provided the mediating, third force between the girls and society.

The group as a system of mutual aid (Schwartz, 1971) was utilized as a process wherein the worker and the group found the common ground between the requirements of group members and those systems they needed to negotiate. Obstacles were identified and challenged in those identified systems. Information, ideas, facts and values were shared by the workers and group members for problem resolution. Workers provided a vision by role modeling and sharing about their own problem solving. Finally, limits and requirements of those systems and the group participants' relationship to them were defined. It was recognized that women, particularly ethnic minority women, encounter more specific and difficult barriers to challenge in order to negotiate in those systems.

### Group Membership/Composition/Formation

An important consideration in the design of prevention programs is when to intervene. Programs intended to prevent adolescent pregnancy, or to motivate adolescents to actively shape their life outcomes, are generally directed toward high school girls. It is not clear just when, in the developmental schema, a girl becomes aware of adult options, but the increasingly early age of adolescent pregnancies suggested that in order to be preventative, the intervention must take place early. The program was directed toward sixth grade girls based on the known increased influence of peers in junior high school.

While group members were quite homogeneous in age, ethnicity, and socioeconomic class, they were not homogeneous in terms of their perception of themselves in relation to life options. One caution in prevention intervention programs is the likelihood of stigmatization resulting from being chosen for prevention of a problem. Since the composition of groups and setting for the work was to be done through public schools, care was taken to include a broad spectrum of girls in the groups and not simply those who were identified as high risk for low perception of control. The composition selection process was that school social workers were asked to identify girls who could benefit from program goals as stated. A caution was given to the school social workers not to just select "potential problem" girls, but a variety of girls. Thus, a heterogeneous factor was introduced into the composition.

Group work literature suggests that a common problem may be the most unifying element in a group (Henry, 1981; Toseland and Rivas, 1984). In these prevention groups, commonality of problem was not easily identified. While the groups were somewhat homogeneous in age, ethnicity, and socioeconomic class, they were more heterogeneous in their perceptions of themselves, their relationships, and future choice making as women. At times, they were diversified by the groups or cliques they hung around with at school, and even by socioeconomic aspirations, or value system. The greatest commonality was the developmental transition of adolescence, ethnic minority status (Black and Hispanic) and lower socioeconomic class.

Groups were convened through the schools, but usually met away from the school premises at a local church or community center. Group size was 8-12 girls and the sessions were 90 minutes long, held once per week. Group workers were social workers or social work students, trained in social group work knowledge and skills.

The beginning group sessions were focused on getting-acquainted activities, development of self and ethnic awareness, and reaching for the common purpose in order to develop a mutually agreed upon contract. Group leadership and other roles emerged early in the group.

## A First Meeting

Most of the 13 girls in the *Foxy Angels* club already knew each other from school. For the ice-breaker exercise, the group workers (Mary, Anglo, MSW group worker, age 33; and Ana, Cuban, BA degree, with group work training, age 22) asked each girl to choose a partner, a person she didn't know very well, and talk about herself for a few minutes, then see how many things each one could remember about the other to relate to the group. They laughed at how these things came out, particularly any information about boyfriends. Shannon said that Tony knew how to get a lot of boyfriends but that she had dumped them all right now.

The purpose of the group had been explained to the girls at a meeting at school when they were asked if they'd like to be in the group. The workers again talked about the commonality of experience of the group members and choice in regards to their lives. Tony said she didn't make any choices, but others started to point out areas in which she does make choices. LaTrayl said, "You always have to make a choice of whether to fight somebody or not.'' Mary said the group has to learn about all the choices they do have to make and how to make some of them, or at least learn some information that would help make them. They all seemed to agree to explore this even though several didn't have much to say about it, or maybe didn't understand it. They seemed to respond more to the idea of learning how to solve problems and agreed they wanted to do that. Shanda said, ''Especially about boys,'' and that brought laughter from all. Ana asked if problems with boys were one of the areas they were all concerned about and there was a lot of head nodding and laughter. The workers agreed this would be an area of focus. Then Mary asked in what other areas they found themselves with problems needing to be solved. Pattie said she fights with her mom a lot; others agreed that problems with parents was an area of concern, and the contracting was underway.

### Doing Together

During the third meeting, we arranged to cook ethnic foods at the center. In preparation for this, we had a lively discussion about what ethnic foods are and how different ethnic foods become popular with ethnic groups. In discussion of what to cook at the center to celebrate their own ethnicity, they decided (for practical reasons mostly) that the easiest thing would be burritos.

At the beginning of the session, while waiting for other members to show up, LaTrayl was discussing her ''encounters'' with the principal and fights between other kids which she has to break up because she is a safety patrol. LaTrayl is aggressive and seems preoccupied with fighting and being tough. She is emerging as leader of the group, seemingly because she is the ''toughest'' girl in the group. While we were waiting, a new girl, Rosilee, came in for the first time to the group. She seemed very self-confident, intelligent and independent. When we began to divide tasks, Rosilee jumped in and began to work and said she knew how to make tortillas.

She wasn't shy even though she knew fewer of the girls than did anyone else. Rosilee's grandparents lived in the neighborhood, not her parents. In fact, her parents had moved out of the projects and were aspiring middle class. Rosilee lived with her grandmother through the week and went to the same school as the other girls in the group.

All the girls were eager to cook and while dividing the jobs, some confusion and arguing emerged over who would do what. At this point, LaTrayl took over. She first asked who wanted to do what and then made assignment decisions, told the others what to do and they did it. Order returned. The cooking all went very well under LaTrayl's able leadership.

In addition to ethnic foods, special holidays and family rituals were brought out, shared and valued in the group. Additional activities were developed under the rubric of the identified social systems. These activities were for the purpose of increasing girls' knowledge and skills in order to better solve problems. Thus, they were viewed as empowerment strategies.

### Health System

Personal body and health system education activities were developed to inform girls about their bodies, and how they function. Sexual activity, contraception, dating and relationships were discussed. In addition, girls were educated about where and how to obtain contraception, advice, physical check-up, and consultation. Field trips were scheduled to the local neighborhood health center to meet actual people in that system. Phone numbers of those people were given to the girls so they would have a face to match with the person they might call. Gynecologists were introduced in an effort to reduce the anxiety about coming to the clinic. Scenarios were presented, role-played, and discussed regarding choices to be made in problem solving around caring for one's body and physical health.

Finally Dr. Ingram arrived. She introduced herself and said she works for Health and Hospitals and was on the TV documentary "13 Million Teenagers" (which dealt with teenage pregnancy). Several girls said they had watched the documentary and asked, "Was it really you?" Dr. Ingram said it was.

Dr. Ingram started by asking the girls about their feelings on being very young and getting pregnant. Sonja adamantly stated, "Don't get pregnant!" Shannon said, "I'd be scared. If you go with a guy and get pregnant and don't know it, then you find out and your mother finds out, then you're in trouble!" When Dr. Ingram asked if they knew how girls got pregnant, they giggled and said, "Yeah, sure." Since they didn't have any questions, Dr. I. suggested they answer some of her questions. This approach dealt gently with their knowledge and lack of it. . . .

Then Dr. I. asked the girls what age they thought was "right" for a girl to have a baby. Shannon said 16; Stacy and Louise, 18. We discussed the pros and cons of having a baby when a person is so young (even 18).

LaTrayl said that if you decide to engage in sexual activity you must also decide on which contraceptive to use in order to avoid an unwanted pregnancy. Dr. I. admitted this seemed a very logical thing to do but many girls she sees never think about this and consequently get pregnant. Shannon asked, "How could a girl get pregnant without 'doing it'?" She was told this is impossible. So Shannon turned to Tony and told her, "You lied to me." According to Tony this had happened to her aunt, but Dr. I. stressed that this was not possible, that she must have had intercourse, and that maybe she had said this in order to avoid getting in trouble with her mom. Tony thought that maybe that's what happened. Again, Dr. I. said there was no way a girl could get pregnant without having sex although many of the pregnant young girls she sees say the same thing.

The girls seemed to like Dr. I. very much. She did a good job of explaining the facts to them, and her way of addressing them seemed to encourage the girls to ask questions. Paula especially asked many questions which certainly interested all of them but that not all felt they could ask. After Dr. I. left, the girls role-played how to handle a situation where a girl must make a decision about having sex. With much laughter and embarrassment, they had fun. We worked directly on the taboo area of sex. The girls left this meeting a lot wiser about their bodies and the choices they must eventually make concerning it.

### Informal Peer Group

This system was chosen due to the heavy reliance of sixth grade girls on their peers for support and as a general reference group. Peer relationships were discussed, and scenarios were presented regarding peer pressure, peer relations and peer support. Problem-solving discussion and role plays were used to educate girls about new ways of handling peer conflict or difficulty. The group itself was an excellent context and means for this component of program activities.

Conflicts arose around traditional vs. non-traditional views of women and what members perceived as appropriate aspirations. In the example group, all girls were from an inner city housing project, except Rosilee who lived part time with her grandmother in the housing project, but whose parents were in the upwardly mobile, lower middle class. She aspired to be a model or a lawyer, a role quite disparate from what most of the girls could see as realistic. She was scapegoated for this break with the culture. A major conflict occurred which resulted in a fistfight between the scapegoated girl and an emerged member-leader in the group.

> An ongoing conflict had been building between Rosilee and some of the other girls, particularly Jackie T., Shonda and Pattie. They seemed to resent her confident manner and her hope for the future. Today we were nearing the ending of the group. We were evaluating the group experience, each one talking about the group. When Rosilee said it had helped her realize how important it is to know that what you want can happen Jackie T. said, "knowing I want to kick your ass is important." Others giggled. Rosilee looked uncomfortable. Mary suggested that Jackie T. talk some more about that, but

Jackie T. declined and her supporters giggled. As the group broke up, Jackie T. was still upset with Rosilee. Rosilee apologized to Jackie T. on the way out of the room, but Jackie T. didn't accept the apology. Several girls were gathering to watch the argument. Apparently Rosilee had called Jackie T. a "bitch" at school. Jackie T. was enticing Rosilee outside so she could "kick her ass." The workers intervened and got the girls into a discussion of what the anger was about—hurt feelings, school gossip. Mary asked each girl how she would like to handle it. Rosilee said she would promise Jackie T. not to say anything to her or about her at school. Jackie T. said that was good, but she still wanted to kick her ass. Ana asked Jackie T. what it would take for her not to want to kick Rosilee's ass. She said, "She'd have to get out of my business at school." Rosilee said, "I will. I told you that." Jackie T. hesitantly replied, "Okay." Mary asked then if it were settled and if they were pleased with the settlement. Both said they were.

Rosilee asked the worker, Mary, for a ride home. As Rosilee and Mary were nearing Mary's car, several girls were following. LaTrayl shoved Rosilee into Jackie T. and fists began flying. With help from a young man nearby, the girls were separated. Upon getting them apart, things looked finished and the tension lowered. Mary said, "I thought we'd worked this out." LaTrayl, the assumed leader of the group, the one who pushed Rosilee into Jackie T., said to Mary, "You don't understand; nothing is settled in the projects until you settle it with your fists." When asked if there was a need to learn alternative ways, Jackie volunteered that talking it out is okay, but here in the projects people expect you to fight it out. Jackie T. appeared to be okay with the settlement previously worked out, but LaTrayl felt it unfinished, and with her leadership position, she called the final shot about how to settle the conflict. The fight seemed to settle, not escalate, the conflict. LaTrayl's style of conflict resolution was very aggressive. She used her leadership position to impose it on the group.

While the group provided an opportunity to look at conflict and learn new ways to handle it, perhaps the culture of the community carried more weight at this moment about how to settle differences. Perhaps, too, Rosilee's new class difference could have been discussed with many levels of consciousness touched. The group did provide new learning in the area. The decision to use those new ways may vary with the girls over time.

Some literature suggests women do not deal with conflict openly in a group (Hagen, 1983). However, conflict is a very common theme in sixth grade adolescent girls and was a prevalent process in these groups. The dynamic process of inclusion/exclusion, typical at this age, was prevalent. The members demonstrated a very open, aggressive style of conflict resolution. This was not easy for the workers, but they did not try to smooth over all conflictual interactions (Henry, 1981), nor did they ignore them. One of the workers' main tasks in the group was the mediation of conflict resolution. The fight came near the ending phase of the group. Fighting or aggression often returns toward the ending of the group. Perhaps this conflict might have been handled differently during the middle phase of the group.

### School and Family

The school system and family system were viewed as places girls have to face problematic situations most frequently. Scenarios reflecting real life school and family problems were presented. Roleplays and discussions were used to educate girls about problem solving at school and at home. Field trips were scheduled to meet counselors, social workers, vice principals—those significant persons who would be important in problem solving at school. Families were invited to meetings where the content of the program was discussed and families were educated about helping girls solve problems at home. Activities were developed to increase girls' abilities to talk to their parents and solicit their help in problem solving.

> The topic for this session was "Difficult Problems at Home." Paula said she hated her step-dad because he was mean to her mom and to her. Pattie said she liked her mother's boyfriend, but she always argued with her mother. Tony said she always fought with her mom about school and housework. She said her mom always wanted her to work around the house and she wanted to be out with her friends. The worker, Mary,

asked if there was some way to work out a deal with her mom — a trade-off. She said, "No, because she won't listen, and we just yell." Mary asked if this is what happens a lot at home, that they can't work out problems with parents because they just argue and yell. Several nodded yes. Mary asked if they'd like to work on learning ways to talk to parents. They said yes. Mary asked Tony to take her mom's role and Mary took hers. Mary modeled ways of negotiation with her mom. Then they switched roles and Tony took her mom's role. Mary asked other girls to take roles of their moms and demonstrate how the situation would be handled. Role-play was used to help girls experience new behaviors and skills for negotiating with parents. They got into it in a real big way, liking the drama and laughing at one another. Tony agreed to go home and try out her new skills. LaTrayl said she knew Tony could do it.

### Career Choice and the Economic System

Educational games and program activities around careers and alternative choices for women were created at a level appropriate for sixth grade girls. Field trips were scheduled to meet ethnically diverse women doing a variety of jobs. Girls were educated about first job seeking and career development. Values clarification exercises were created around career and life options. One important game was a life option's bidding game wherein girls had to choose which life option on which to bid: marriage, house, car, status in community, job, clothes, jewelry, opportunity to serve others, making the world a better place, business operator.

Each girl was given a sheet with instructions and the list of items to bid on. They were instructed that they could bid on everything or nothing, but that this was their big opportunity to bid on those things they really wanted. The highest bid went for a car, $80 by Shannon. The next highest bid was made by Pattie for $75 to have close friends. Paula bought the marriage for $50 and Rosilee bought travel opportunity for $45. The rest of the items were more or less equally divided among the girls and bought with bids ranging from $5 to $15. After some initial confusion, the girls really got into the game and on the second and third rounds were maneuvering to see who had how much money left, running up the cost of items so there would be no more money left to be bid on the item they wanted. Shanda, LaTrayl and Sonja entered a cooperative arrangement where they pooled resources and jointly bought items to share. Then Paula suggested they make up their own items. Added items included adopting a child, having a good boy friend, being president of the United States, going to Africa, owning a bank. They laughed and had great fun with this game. It also had great potential for consciousness raising and opening options.

### Attendance, Norm Development and Cohesion

Attendance was always high at meetings. The girls seemed to view group membership as a privilege. Field trips related to group content and reward helped to keep group membership highly valued. Cohesion and norm development did not occur rapidly. Group norms modeled by workers (Henry, 1981) eventually evolved in the group around behaviors such as not siding against each other during group and letting each person talk without interruption or put-down. A norm evolved that suggested that members had to take active roles in solving their own problems. Cohesion occurred over time with the experience of interaction and conflict resolution.

### Evaluation

The program was initially directed toward inner city ethnic minority girls and was later expanded to non-inner city, non-ethnic group schools as well. An evaluation was done on the program as a whole. This empowerment project which began in 1979 was evaluated after one and one-half years utilizing pre- and post-measures to compare program participants and control group girls who had not participated in the program. The control groups were selected by either random assignment of those girls selected by social workers to participate in the program into a control group, or by choosing one sixth grade class in a neighborhood for the program, and another for control group testing. Pre- and post-testing was done before and after the program to determine differences both pre-intervention and post-intervention. Measures consisted of the Nowicki-Strickland and Internal-External Control Scale for females (1973), and a values checklist. No differences were found on the internality-externality perception of control measures between participants and control girls. However, participants were found to have significantly changed their value orientations toward less traditional women's values regarding career options, whereas the control group girls did not (Simmons and Parsons, 1983a).

Results of that evaluation suggested a format change for the program: an increase from 12 weeks, the initial intervention time period, to 24 weeks and greater emphasis on action oriented programming. This is consistent with the time needed for group norms, roles and cohesion to develop. A subsequent evaluation of the program was conducted in 1982 on program participants from working class socioeconomic backgrounds and participants from socioeconomic backgrounds below the poverty line, and a control group of nonparticipants from working class backgrounds. Measures included Connell's Multidimensional Measure of Children's Perceptions of Control (1985) in areas of school, social relationships and general life events, and Harter's Perceived Competence Scale for Children (1982). Additionally, knowledge of and interest in traditional and non-traditional careers for women were tested. Results showed an increase in internality on all three dimensions of Connell's scale for the working class participants, but not for the control group, and no differences for girls from poverty backgrounds. Participants from working class backgrounds also showed significant increases in perceived competence for school achievement and general competence, but a decrease in perceived competence was found for poverty background girls. Finally, participants from working class backgrounds were found to know about more careers, both traditional and non-traditional, at the end of the program; however, that finding did not hold for girls from poverty backgrounds (Simmons and Parsons, 1983b).

The poverty background girls actually had pre-tested higher on internality than the working class girls, which was not predicted. After completion of the program, their internality decreased. The higher pre-test score could be attributed to tough street-smart kids as a reference group on the pre-test, with perhaps a change in reference groups on the post-test. The program content and format may not have empowered girls who were unable to bridge the distance between their own lives and those knowledge and skills encountered in the program. This indicates a need for workers to learn more about how to reach the poorest children and how to mediate effectively for actual resources that may increase a sense of hope and power, lowering the sense of fatalism.

Interestingly, the evaluation showed that black girls in the program changed more than any other ethnic group. Group workers' perceptions were that those groups which were more successful were those wherein they were able to resolve conflict and build group cohesion. Group workers observed that in the groups of girls from the school in a poverty area, conflict resolution was less successful, and the level of cohesion was low compared to other groups from working class neighborhoods.

## *CONCLUSION*

This group program was implemented with purposes and goals to increase girls' self-esteem, perceptions of control over their lives, and their knowledge regarding role alternatives for women. The goals were considered appropriate for a prevention program for disempowered girls. Caution was used concerning further stereotyping and stigmatizing girls who would participate in the program.

Empowerment was used as an intervention framework and the mutual aid of the small group was used as a method. Activities were developed to increase knowledge and skills for problem solving in four major social systems which were thought to be relevant areas in the girls' lives. Activities focused on education, discussion, role-play and firsthand learning about access to problem-solving resources in those specified areas. The development of mutual aid in the group was the primary means for change to occur.

Evaluation showed that girls' value systems changed from more traditional to less traditional, and for working class girls, an increase in knowledge regarding role alternatives for women and an increase in perception of control were realized. Further study is needed to determine if fatalistic attitudes of externality are a major factor in adolescent pregnancy, and if using groups to increase girls' problem-solving abilities and systems negotiation skills indeed affect their perceptions that they can control events in their lives. An increased activity level of worker mediation in the environment to actually obtain resources for and with the poorest girls and their families and communities may also be critically important in providing the external motivation for a positive perception of power and alternatives.

## REFERENCES

Connell, J.P. "A New Multidimensional Measure of Children's Perceptions of Control." *Child Development* 56(2), 1985, pp. 1018-1041.

Findley, M., and H.M. Cooper. "Locus of Control and Academic Achievement: A Literature Review." *Journal of Personality and Social Psychology* 44(2), pp. 419-427.

Garvin, C. *Contemporary Group Work*. 2nd edition. Englewood Cliffs, NJ: Prentice Hall, 1987.

Gitterman, A. "The School: Group Work in the Public Schools" in W. Schwartz and S. Zalba, eds. *The Practice of Group Work*. New York: Columbia University Press, 1971, p. 48.

Gitterman, A., and L. Shulman, eds. *Mutual Aid Groups and the Life Cycle*. Itasca, IL: Peacock Publishers, 1986, p. 3.

Hagen, B.H. "Managing Conflict in All-Women Groups." *Social Work With Groups* 6(3/4), 1983, pp. 95-103.

Harter, S.A. "The Perceived Competence Scale for Children." *Child Development* 53(3), 1982, pp. 87-97.

Hartford, M. *Groups in Social Work*. New York: Columbia University Press, 1971, p. 34.

Henry, S. *Group Skills in Social Work*. Itasca, IL: F. E. Peacock Publishing, Inc. 1981, p. 60.

Lee, J. "No Place to Go: Homeless Women" in A. Gitterman and L. Shulman, eds. *Mutual Aid and the Life Cycle*. Itasca, IL: Peacock Publishers, 1986, p. 246.

Lieberman, J.J. "Locus of Control as Related to Birth Control Knowledge, Attitudes and Practices." *Adolescence* 16(61), 1981, pp. 1-10.

Nowicki, S., B. Strickland, Jr. "A Locus of Control Scale for Children." *Journal of Consulting and Clinical Psychology* 40(2) 1973, pp. 148-155.

Robbins, C., H.B. Kaplan, and S.S. Martin. "Antecedents of Pregnancy Among Unmarried Adolescents." *Journal of Marriage and the Family*, August 1985, pp. 576-583.

Ross, S. *The Youth Values Project*. New York: The Population Institute, 1979.

Rotter, J.B. "Generalized Expectancies for Internal versus External Control of Reinforcement." *Psychological Monographs*, 80(1), 1966.

Ryan, W. *Blaming the Victim*. New York: Random House, 1972.

Scales, P. "The Context of Sex Education and Reduction of Teenage Pregnancy." *Child Welfare* 58(4), 1979, pp. 263-273.

Schwartz, W., and S. Zalba, eds. *The Practice of Group Work*. New York: Columbia University Press, 1976, pp. 1-24.

Sherman, L. "Development of Children's Perception of Internal Locus of Control: A Cross-Sectional and Longitudinal Analysis." *Journal of Personality*. 52(4), 1984, pp. 338-354.

Simmons, C.H., and R.J. Parsons. "Empowerment for Role Alternatives in Adolescence." *Adolescence* 27(69), 1983, pp. 196-198.

Simmons, C.H., and R.J. Parsons. "Developing Internality and Perceived Competence: The Empowerment of Adolescent Girls." *Adolescence* 28(72), 1983, pp. 917-922.

Solomon, B. *Black Empowerment: Social Work in Oppressed Communities*. New York: Columbia University Press, 1976.

Toseland, R., and R. Rivas. *An Introduction to Group Work Practice*. New York: McMillan Publishing Co., 1984, pp. 124-125.

Young, R. "Vocational Choice and Values in Adolescent Women." *Sex Roles* 10(7-8), 1984, p. 489.

# The Need for Mutual-Aid Groups in a Drop-In for Homeless Women: The *Sistering* Case

Margot Breton

**SUMMARY.** *Sistering* is a Toronto city drop-in which serves a diverse population of transient and homeless women, all of whom are oppressed by the "feminization of poverty." This article reviews the nurturing/educating approach which underlies the drop-in program. It raises a number of issues related to this approach, and considers the need for structure and for effective integration of small mutual-aid groups within drop-in services to oppressed populations.

## *INTRODUCTION*

*Sistering* is a Toronto city drop-in which serves transient and homeless women. It is housed in a community centre, relatively close to downtown and to the city's hostels, and is easily accessible by public transportation. It is funded 70% by the Ontario Ministry of Health, 20% by United Way, 5% by the Municipality of Toronto, and the rest by memberships and donations.

Many of the women who use *Sistering* (more than 50%) are chronic or ex-psychiatric patients, a number are older women who have lost their homes through widowhood, separation or hospitalization of a spouse, while others are unemployed young or middle-aged women. Though the women come from a wide variety of backgrounds and situations, all can be identified in some way or

Margot Breton, MSW, is Associate Professor on the Faculty of Social Work, University of Toronto, 246 Bloor Street West, Toronto, Ontario M5S 1A1 Canada.

other as victimized and oppressed — all are subject to forces out of their control. Those who have experienced psychiatric illnesses and are now back on the street are victims of inadequate or poorly supported deinstitutionalization programs; they and most of the other users of *Sistering* are victims of the crisis in low-cost urban housing and of alienating and punitive welfare policies (for example, the requirement of having a permanent address in order to quality for welfare); finally all are victims of the feminization of poverty.

As *Sistering* tries to help these women to overcome the effects of their victimization, it faces the dilemma that in dealing with oppressed people, it is easy to try to compensate for their victimization in a paternalistic manner that creates further helplessness. It is easy to oppress the oppressed by seeing them only as victims, and not as whole persons, thereby stigmatizing them instead of collaborating towards their empowerment. It must be acknowledged that the empowerment of oppressed people is a complex process. On the one hand, one must guard against false empowerment, or against pretending that environments can always be manipulated in one's favor. On the other hand, one cannot settle for less than doing whatever it is possible to do.

This article reviews the nurturing/educating approach which underlies the *Sistering* drop-in program, and raises a number of issues related to this approach. It then considers the need for structure and for an effective integration of small groups within drop-in services.

## THE NURTURING/EDUCATING PARADIGM

The *Sistering* drop-in was planned and developed as a "refuge for rest and recuperation" (Caplan, 1974) but also as a socialization to competence and maintenance of competence milieu (Breton, 1984). It was assumed that to create this milieu, nurturing and educating elements would need to be programmed into the service offered. Nurturing was seen as providing opportunities for people to develop or maintain positive coping attitudes, such as attitudes of hope and trust, while educating would provide opportunities to learn and/or to practice the cognitive and behavioral skills for coping, such as problem-solving and observing rules of social behavior. It was further assumed that for the nurturing and educating opportunities to be productive, the drop-in would need to present its users with optimal challenges (Harter, 1978), i.e., with expectations that were neither too high nor too low. This remains a formidable task, for while it is imperative to respect the idea of an informal and non-intrusive drop-in centre, where women are free to come and go as they please, the long-range goal of promoting and maintaining competence cannot survive unless the program encourages a learning and consciousness-raising process which will enable its users to eventually have more control over their lives.

This is not meant to infer that the homeless women who use *Sistering* would see their situation change immediately if only they learned how to use the system or how to problem-solve. Much of their plight is due to socioeconomic circumstances pitted against which the best individual coping skills will fail. As Stoner (1983) remarks: "Homeless women do not choose their circumstances. They are victims of forces over which they have lost control." It is precisely to give back some measure of control to these women that *Sistering* strives to be a nurturing/educating milieu which provides optimal challenges to its users.

## *Nurturing*

To nurture means to meet basic human needs for physical comfort, food and shelter and higher level needs for a sense of belonging, for self-esteem and for self-actualization (Maslow, 1954). For homeless women who must be out of the hostels during the daytime (which is the general rule), the drop-in provides a roof over their heads, a warm, clean and dry place to sit and rest their feet without getting hassled, and a space where they can sleep if they have been walking all night, or if the noise, the crowding and the stealing which regularly goes on in some of the hostels have kept them awake. Some food is provided: there is a constant supply of coffee, tea and soup supplied by a local merchant since the beginning of the program. Physical comfort comes in the guise of access to showers (the staff keep a clean supply of towels and soap) and to laundry facilities; it also comes through hairdressing and through make-up sessions, both of which were provided by the staff initially, but are now the responsibility of professionals who weekly donate time to the program; these are highly appreciated features of the drop-in. Finally, physical nurturing includes the safe-keeping and administering of medication to some of the more disoriented women who come regularly to the drop-in (the staff have established close relationships with doctors, nurses and social workers in various mental health and hospital clinics as well as with a number of doctors and dentists who are willing to deal with poor patients).

In terms of meeting the higher level needs, nurturing becomes more complex. A casual observer of the drop-in would conclude that its users feel "at home" in the *Sistering* room. The nonbureaucratic aspect of the service, the fact, for example, that a woman who walks in for the first time will be warmly welcomed, offered a cup of coffee or tea, but not required to give her name or to submit to an intake interview, gives that woman an immediate sense of belonging and of being on her own turf, not on someone else's. Furthermore, this fundamentally nonjudgmental approach extends to accepting the fact that some women will do nothing but sit alone for hours, drink coffee, smoke, and then leave. It cannot be over-emphasized that allowing the women to choose how they use the drop-in is, in itself, empowering.

The problem, however, is deciding if the women who signal that they do not want to talk or participate in an activity are choosing to be left alone. It would appear more realistic to assume that, while they may want to be alone some of the time, many, if not most, have such good reasons not to trust people, and so few skills in relating to people, that without specific and repeated efforts to reach them they will remain uninvolved (Breton, 1985; Brooks, 1978). Therefore, unless there are efficient outreach efforts to the many seemingly passive users of the drop-in, the nurturing aspects of the program will simply feed into the "helplessness training" (Brown, 1981) with which so many women are burdened.

Developing and/or maintaining a sense of self-esteem when one is living on the street, in a hostel or a dingy rooming house is not easy. The staff attempt to be supportive by listening to the women, directing them to the various services they are entitled to, and helping them to become aware of and to insist on their rights — the stuff of consciousness-raising and of assertiveness-training. Practitioners who have worked with victims have identified the need to begin by encouraging this kind of self-focus, for: "Autonomy and a sense of powerfulness begin when a woman is willing to examine her own issues, feelings and behavior. This often represents a change in life-long patterns of other directedness and dependence." (Hartman, 1983).

Unfortunately, the differences among the women and the range of their attitudes and abilities is such that, whereas a small mutual-aid group with a consciousness-raising focus would enhance the development and maintenance of self-esteem most effectively, the paraprofessional staff have found it simpler to help the women individually. This raises an important issue, for providing only individual help to oppressed people whose problems are of a class nature (and such are the feminization of poverty and the inadequate deinstitutionalization of chronic psychiatric patients) is, in the long run, counterproductive. A more radical, political stance is needed. When people are oppressed, what is necessary is their liberation from oppression. And "liberation implies a break with the status-quo . . . it calls for a social revolution" (Gutierrez, 1986). This leads to a question which is at the heart of social group work practice with oppressed people: "How can programs meet immediate individual needs and at the same time constitute steps towards the building of a more just society?" In terms of a drop-in for homeless women, part of the answer lies in the systematic use of mutual-aid, consciousness-raising groups. This issue will be addressed in a later section.

### Educating/Challenging

The decision to locate *Sistering* is a community centre was made purposefully so that the drop-in would "be perceived as part of the normal recreational-educational programs serving normal residents of a community (versus a physically separate and segregated space which might be seen as catering only to the needs of an abnormal population)" (Breton, 1984). This normalization stance automatically introduced educating and challenging aspects into the program, principally in the form of a demand to follow some basic rules of social behavior. After a short trial-and-error period, it was established that there would be no physical fights and no prolonged screaming and carrying-on: definite time-limits now exist for "blowing-up," and consequences of refusing to conform to behavioral expectations are enforced, albeit with compassion – the women have to leave the room and the Centre temporarily. This has seemed to work well, as "even the most disturbed women have discovered that to enjoy the benefits of the drop-in, they have to comply with these basic rules of social conduct, and they do" (Breton, 1984). A "no stealing" rule had to be introduced early on, also entailing temporary banishment; this rule has not worked as well as the other, and stealing still goes on.

In spite of this, mutual trust has been growing between the staff and the women, who are increasingly challenged to participate in the running of the drop-in. This is a crucial issue, for "the self-help process combats learned helplessness by empowering its' members" (Hartman, 1983). As Latin American liberation theologians, who have been struggling for years to empower some of the poorest and most oppressed people in the world, insist: "the process of liberation requires the active participation of the oppressed" (Gutierrez, 1986). This participation will vary according to abilities. In the case of the women who come to *Sistering*, it may mean helping to keep the room tidy, or bringing the more disoriented women to doctors' appointments or to look for rooming houses. It can also mean participating in an International Woman's Day rally, either indirectly through sewing a huge banner carried during rallies (and which now adorns a wall in the *Sistering* room) or directly by actually attending and marching. A development which attests to the "maturing" of the program was the formation, a few years ago, of a volunteers' group made up of long-term *Sistering* users.

Other elements of education and challenge are introduced through special programs. Doctors and public health nurses have held small group discussions on birth control, the proper use of medication, the dangers of street drugs, and on other topics; nutritionists have talked about nutrition on welfare budgets; and life-skills teachers have demonstrated low-budget, roominghouse, hot-plate cooking. As homelessness escalates, *Sistering* is introducing a series of regular monthly meetings with a specialist who will discuss with the women strategies for securing housing. Trips to art galleries, science centres, parks, and other points of interest continue to open horizons and challenge the women to learn about the urban resources available to them.

Finally, recognizing that the qualities of the environment which induce growth include feedback on behavior (Germain, 1981), and acknowledging that police officers are a major element in the environment of transient and homeless women, the local police were encouraged from the start to drop in for a cup of coffee and a chat. They have become "regulars": they play cards with the women, help out when someone is seriously ill and must be rushed to the hospital (which happens often), now and then host a lunch (they prepare and serve all the food), and also have "long and serious, though informal, discussions with the women on issues such as loitering, police tactics re: 'keeping the peace,' and behaviors which constitute a public disturbance" (Breton, 1984). These rational discussions and nonconfrontative encounters have challenged the women's perception of the police as just some of the many people who harass them, and have helped significantly the integration of the women in the community.

The "normalization" option has its costs, one of which is that the use of discipline, or the challenge to the women to bear the consequences of their behavior, could mean that *Sistering* loses the most alienated and needy of the women it wants to serve. This happens infrequently; in most cases, the women who cannot manage the rules of the drop-in are severely mentally disturbed and *Sistering* then acts as a diagnostic facility which periodically concludes that a woman cannot cope outside of a psychiatric institution at that point.

A more central issue is to ensure that the educating-challenging part of the program is a response to the women's needs, not a response to the administrators' (the Board members and indirectly the government bureaucrats responsible for funding the drop-in) need of proofs of the efficacy of the service offered. "Proofs" in the area of delivery of psychosocial services are notoriously difficult to establish, and the temptation to avoid the difficulty by concentrating on the professional legitimacy of the services themselves (i.e., concentrating on input not on output) is also notorious and results, often, in a push for therapeutic, clinical or educational professional services even though they are not always necessary. This has led to another dilemma for *Sistering*. The paraprofessional staff have an impressive capacity to reach the women, to establish trusting relationships and to serve as models. Moreover, many of the services the women need do not require professional training. However, a professional social group worker could bring to the program an ability to identify those needs which are best met through specialized small group services. Keeping in mind that the oppressed "must be the primary agents of their own liberation" (Boff and Boff, 1986), the group worker, the paraprofessional staff and representatives of the women who come to the drop-in (perhaps some members of the volunteers' group, and others who might surprise everyone with their willingness to participate) would then get together and translate this identification of need into effective programming. Though this kind of program planning has taken place, *Sistering* is still searching for the optimal way of integrating professional and non-professional services (Breton, 1986), and of ensuring the active participation of the women in the planning of programs.

A related issue concerns services to the deinstitutionalized. Lamb (1981) has argued that in regard to a large number of psychiatric patients, insistence on rehabilitation may only reflect society's "disapproval of dependency, inactivity and acceptance of public support." Some mentally-impaired women who come to *Sistering* will always remain more dependent, more inactive and in greater need of support than the rest of the women — in other words, some cannot but rely more heavily on the nurturing component of the program. Services (like *Sistering*) whose focus in on building and maintaining competence must recognize these realities. They must recognize as well that even the people who can take advantage of challenges will need support in their quest for empowerment. Oppressed people not only need to learn to provoke changes in the systems that affect them; their efforts at bringing about changes must be supplemented by external interventions (Tucker, 1984) whenever the power to impact these systems lies with people other than the oppressed themselves.

*Sistering*'s nurturing/educating paradigm has proven an effective response to the needs of low-income, homeless and lonely women. Support for the program from the Toronto mental health and social welfare communities (both at the professional and paraprofessional levels) has been such that a recent research concluded that a satellite drop-in program should be opened in another part of the city, and the *Sistering II* drop-in is now in operation. However, the paradigm itself raises some contentious issues: (1) increased helplessness as a possible by-product of nurturing; (2) focusing on individual help when problems are of a class nature; (3) paternalistic or "mothering" versus "sistering" approaches to education; (4) integrating professional and paraprofessional services; and (5) the need for external support of empowerment.

The next section will argue that to deal effectively with these issues, a nurturing/educating paradigm must include structured mutual-aid groups in which consciousness-raising (or political awareness) is developed.

## THE NEED FOR STRUCTURE
## VIA MUTUAL-AID GROUPS

It would be inconsistent, indeed absurd, to have a completely structured drop-in: by nature, such a service is consumer-determined and therefore must allow maximum program flexibility. When *Sistering* was set up, it was recognized that respecting the liberal nature of a drop-in, while at the same time encouraging a learning process presented a challenge. After roughly six years of operation, one can say that *Sistering* has met this challenge fairly well, and that this has been due in part to the introduction of structure into the program. Structure in this context means "a deliberately employed vehicle for creating, in microcosm, particular social situations for learning purposes" (Middleman and Goldberg, 1972).

Introducing structure into a drop-in service is not always easy. At one point in time, it was as though the staff of *Sistering*, and the program, had been "sucked into" the improvisational style of living of the transient and homeless women who come to the drop-in (just as a family worker can get sucked into a dysfunctional family system). The need for more structure and more learning opportunities — for more competence-building — which board members advocated became one of the earliest points of dissention between they and the staff. It was difficult for the latter to accept that a drop-in could allow for a programmatic mix of small groups, mass activities, "free" or totally unstructured time, and individual crisis intervention. The staff frankly believed that the nurturing aspect of the nurturing/educating paradigm was of much greater value to the women than the educating aspect; perceiving nurturing as their function, they strongly opposed mutual-aid groups.

One of the major reasons for their opposition to mutual-aid groups was their own sense of being overwhelmed by the seemingly insurmountable problems facing the homeless. This feeling of powerlessness, to which Lee (1987) has referred in her analysis of social work with oppressed populations, can lead to the implicit assumption that inviting homeless women to join a small mutual-aid, consciousness-raising group will only produce sterile discussions of problems. The staff of *Sistering* has been torn between the desire to see the users of the drop-in get a better deal and the determination not to set the women up for failure. They seem to be wary of the possible pitfalls of "talking help" to oppressed people, perhaps sensing that: "Never shall we attain to real liberation merely by fostering 'aspirations' to the same — anymore than we shall feed the hungry by reading kitchen recipes to them" (Boff and Boff, 1986). This dilemma is compounded with the paraprofessional staff's inexperience of social group work and their suspicions about "therapy" — not that these suspicions are entirely unfounded: oppressed women have often been doubly victimized through the intervention of psychiatry acting as "the subtle hand-maiden of the status-quo" (Eastman, 1973). Moreover, when one looks at the proliferation of "treatment groups" in social work, and at the increasing number of social workers defining themselves as "therapists," one understands how paraprofessionals would assume that social work groups would be no different than psychiatrist-led therapy groups.

While all this is true, it is possible to identify a number of clear and valid purposes on the basis of which small mutual-aid groups for homeless women could be convened in the context of a drop-in service. For example, homeless women generally need better information on health resources and on their rights to access these resources; and they especially need to learn how to use these resources, for "research (McDonald and Piliavin, 1981) indicates that, when people are unfamiliar with, and therefore inexperienced in the use of services, even 'strong' knowledge manipulation, i.e., providing large and varied amounts of information on services, does not result in increased use of these services'' (Breton, 1985). A small group whose purpose would be to help the women to take advantage of health facilities would go a long way in preventing or alleviating some of the more painful physical conditions many homeless women unnecessarily endure. The "strength in numbers" phenomenon strongly suggests that groups will be more effective than individual counselling in enabling oppressed and homeless women to develop the attitudes and skills necessary to face the daunting task of dealing with the bureaucracy of health. Furthermore, where services are lacking and the rights of the women to medical and dental care are denied, groups that foster political awareness can lead to effective social action. At *Sistering* a beginning was made in this direction through the formation of a short-term group in which a social worker helped some of the women to deal primarily with health-related issues, culminating in the production of a reference manual listing sympathetic public clinics and doctors and dentists willing to take poor patients. Though the group focused on health, the problem of accessing relatively decent housing was also addressed. Community resource persons were invited on three occasions: the first two guests were representatives of support services, the third was the Housing Coordinator for Welfare. At the meeting with the Coordinator, the ambiguities of eligibility to public housing were vigorously debated, and the women briefly considered the possibility of writing letters to appropriate bodies on whether or not they had rights to appeal these determinations. As this was the second to last session of the short-term group, the possibility was not pursued. However, given the interest and the resolve the group demonstrated, it is not unreasonable to assume that a long-term group could have developed as a consciousness-raising mutual-aid group taking social action on issues such as housing rights.

Another group with a clear purpose could be a poetry group modelled on the group for emotionally isolated men described by Bresler (1982): many homeless women have had to "toughen themselves" to live on the street and have become emotionally isolated in order to survive; such a group could help them to share their concerns, fears and hopes, and thus serve to mitigate their emotional isolation. For those isolated women who would not join a poetry group, another group could model itself, to some extent, on Joyce and Hazelton's (1982) group for women recovering from alcoholism and other addictions. This group could have as a clear purpose to teach the women to form meaningful relationships outside the family. Many users of *Sistering* suffer from being cut-off from their families and from the nurturing roles they used to play or have longed to play. This group could teach them "alternatives to the socially approved nurturing role within the family," using co-leaders to "model supportive relationships between women," and to establish "group norms and values that would not limit or influence its female members to adhere to stereotypic feminine roles and behaviours (i.e., emotionally passive, dependent, submissive, powerless)" (Joyce and Hazelton, 1982).

Furthermore, one of the purposes of Joyce and Hazelton's groups was to help members to collectively identify strengths and goals. This purpose is relevant to oppressed homeless women, e.g., to collectively identify the goal of lobbying for needed housing, and so particularly is one of the methods they used, which was to focus on the "critical periods" of women's lives as outlined in Scarf's *Unfinished Business* (1980). This approach would be very productive with the users of *Sistering*, and other drop-ins for oppressed women, provided it acted as a consciousness-raising mechanism leading to some action — not merely to deeper insight into their situations. Last but not least, there could be a group (or groups) whose purpose would be pure pleasure, fun, enjoyment and mutual support: such groups could make more effective use of the space available in the community centre. The right to have fun and to enjoy life may be one of the least-recognized rights denied to oppressed people. There is no dearth of potentially meaningful and clear purposes for groups within drop-ins such as *Sistering*. Identifying and prioritizing these purposes becomes part of giving a competence-promoting structure to drop-in programs.

Once purposes have been identified and prioritized by all concerned, the next step is to ensure that groups will make effective use of activities, mindful that: "If we continue to extend group work practice to persons with special needs, reclaiming and extending

our use of activities as an important change strategy is essential"
(Gentry, 1984). In working with oppressed people, this means dis-
covering or being sensitive to how intra-group activities can lead to
extra-group action. The essence of competence is that one has some
control over one's environment — that one can have some impact on
(or one can change) one's environment. In terms of social group
work practice, an important start is to promote mutual-aid within a
small group, for having an impact on people in one's immediate
environment can lead to a sense of power and of competence.

However, mutual-aid must be perceived and promoted as an empowering mechanism, *not* as a therapeutic condition. Granted that
mutual-aid always has a personally beneficial effect ("therapeutic"
if one wants to call it so), in work with oppressed people, it is
morally perverse to focus on the personal and neglect the political.
This does not imply that as soon as a group is convened, the worker
will get members to write to their member of parliament or their
congressmen/congresswomen. It means (as all liberation theorists
insist) that one fosters an awareness of the non-personal dimension
of problems at the same time as one is receptive to immediate concerns and needs.

It may be that if group workers ally themselves to oppressed populations, they will simply have to abandon the luxury of forever
dichotomizing between "social action groups" and other types of
groups. All their work will have to involve a struggle for a more just
society, and in all their work, they will need to apply "the skills of
social action group work" (Lee, 1988). Furthermore the struggle
for a just society cannot take place exclusively within the confines
of the small group — it must transcend it and involve action in and
on the environing social systems.

## CONCLUSION

This paper emphasizes the importance of introducing structure,
through the use of small groups, into a drop-in for homeless women
in order to provide an optimal balance of nurturing and learning
experiences. It cautions that the nurturing aspects of services such
as the *Sistering* drop-in could further victimize oppressed women
by generating helplessness, while the educating/challenging part of

the program could be seen as putting the responsibility solely on the individual homeless woman to change her situation, in effect stating that it is up to her alone to get out of the trap of homelessness.

Competence-building and competence-maintaining programs nurture in a fashion that strengthens, and educate and challenge in a fashion that mutually raises the consciousness of all involved. Such programs create opportunities for true empowerment.

## REFERENCES

Boff, L. and Boff, C. *Liberation Theology: From Confrontation to Dialogue*. San Francisco: Harper and Row, 1986, 31, 53.

Bresler, E. "Filling an Empty Universe: Poetry Therapy with a Group of Emotionally Isolated Men," *Social Work with Groups*, 1982, 5 (3), 65-70.

Breton, M. "A Drop-In for Transient Women: Using the Physical Environment to Promote Competence," *Social Work*, Vol. 29 (6) Nov./Dec. 1984, 542-545.

Breton, M. "Reaching and Engaging People: Issues and Practice Principles," *Social Work with Groups*, Vol. 8 (3). Fall 1985, 7-21.

Breton, M. "Professional Group Work Practice with the Hard-to-Reach in Paraprofessional/Community Based Settings," Unpublished, 11.

Brooks, A. "Group Work on the Bowery," *Social Work with Groups*, 1978, 1 (1), 53-63.

Brown, P. "Women and Competence," in A.N. Maluccio (ed.), *Promoting Competence in Clients: A New/Old Approach to Social Work Practice*, New York: The Free Press, 1981.

Caplan, G. *Support Systems and Community Mental Health*. New York: Behavioural Publications, 1974, 6.

Eastman, P. "Consciousness-Raising as a Resocialization Process for Women," *Smith College Studies in Social Work*, XLIII, (June, 1973), 153-183.

Gentry, M.E. "Developments in Activity Analysis: Recreation and Group Work Revisited," *Social Work with Groups*, 1984, 7 (1), 35-44.

Germain, C.B. "The Physical Environment and Social Work Practice," in A.N. Maluccio (ed.), *Promoting Competence in Clients: A New/Old Approach to Social Work Practice*, New York: The Free Press, 1981.

Gutierrez, J. *A Theology of Liberation*. Maryknoll, N.J.: Orbis Books, 1986, 102-113.

Harter, S. "Effectance Motivation Reconsidered: Toward a Developmental Model," *Human Development*, 1978, 21, 34-64.

Hartman, S. "A Self-Help Group for Women in Abusive Relationships," *Social Work with Groups*, 1983, 5: (3/4), 133-146.

Joyce, C. and Hazelton, P. "Women in Groups: A Pre-Group Experience for Women in Recovery from Alcoholism and Other Addictions," *Social Work with Groups*, 1982, 5 (1), 57-63.

Lamb, H.R. "What Did We Really Expect from Deinstitutionalization?," *Hospital and Community Psychiatry*, 1981, 32 (2), 105-109.

Lee, J.A.B. "Social Work with Oppressed Populations: Jane Addams Won't You Please Come Home?," *Social Group Work: Competence and Values in Practice*, Joseph Lassner, Kathleen Powell and Elaine Finnegan, Eds., Monographic Supplement #2, Vol. 10, 1987: 1-16.

Lee, J.A.B. Personal Communication, 1988.

Maslow, A.H. *Motivation and Personality*. New York: Harper and Row, 1954.

McDonald, T.P. and Piliavin, I. "Impact of Separation on Community Social Service Utilization," *Social Service Review*, 1981, 55 (4), 528-535.

Middleman, R. and Goldberg, G. "The Concept of Structure in Experiential Learning," *The 1972 Annual Handbook for Group Facilitators*, Iowa City, Iowa: University Associates, 1972, 203-210.

Scarf, M. *Unfinished Business: Pressure Points in the Lives of Women*. New York: Doubleday, 1980.

Stoner, M.R. "The Plight of Homeless Women," *Social Service Review*, 1983, 555-581.

Tucker, S. "Minority Issues in Community Mental Health," in B. Compton and B. Galaway (eds.), *Social Work Processes*, 3rd edition, 1984, 167-175.

# Group Development
# and Shared Decision Making
# Working with Homeless
# Mentally Ill Women

Toby Berman-Rossi
Marcia B. Cohen

**SUMMARY.** An on-site Community Support System (CSS) team in a single room occupancy (SRO) hotel worked with homeless mentally ill residents toward rehabilitation through empowerment. The issue of power in the group process over a five-year period of time is described and analyzed.

## *INTRODUCTION*

In the past few years, as the service needs of the homeless mentally ill have become more visible, social workers have been asked to develop practice competence in working with this extremely disadvantaged and very challenging population. Unfortunately, there has been little literature on practice with homeless mentally ill clients to assist social workers in their skill development. Available material has primarily focused upon: the characteristics of the population (Baxter and Hopper, 1981; Arce, 1983; Morse, 1984; Roth, 1985; Rossi et al., 1987), their needs (Martin, 1982; Lipton et al., 1983; Stoner, 1983; Cohen et al., 1984; Golden, 1986) and the fragmentation of needed services (Bachrach, 1984; Lamb, 1984;

Toby Berman-Rossi, DSW, is Assistant Professor in the Columbia University School of Social Work, and Marcia B. Cohen, PhD, is affiliated with Columbia University Community Services and is Lecturer in the Columbia University School of Social Work, McVickar, 622 West 113th Street, New York, NY 10025.

Bachrach, 1985; Levine and Stockdill, 1986). Writings on practice with this population have concentrated on the skills of providing individual services (Levine, 1984; Cohen, 1985; Putnam, et al., 1986). Discussion of the skills of working with this population in groups is practically nonexistent. This neglect is particularly striking when we consider that group services are at the core of many programs serving the homeless mentally ill. The works of Lee (1986) and Shapiro (1971a; 1971b) are notable exceptions. They address the kind of alienation and disaffiliation which characterize life on the streets and point to the ways in which group services provide a primary means of increasing connectedness as well as experience of competence.

## CLIENT CHARACTERISTICS

Homeless mentally ill women comprise a significant portion of the homeless population. According to a recent estimate (U.S. Dept. of Health and Human Services, 1984) it is suggested that women comprise between 15 and 30% of the homeless population. Some researchers have found mental illness to be more prevalent among homeless women than among homeless men (Shulman, 1981; Crystal, 1984; Bachrach, 1985). Estimates of the extent of mental illness in the homeless population vary widely, with most estimates falling between 20 and 50% (Hopper and Hamburg, 1984).

These statistics do not convey the pain of oppressed, disenfranchised, alienated people. Social isolation, limited power over the environment, and a high degree of interpersonal and daily living stressors are the norm (Bahr and Garrett, 1976; Rose and Black, 1985; Cohen, 1988). The day to day existence of homeless mentally ill women abound with experiences of loss and there is growing evidence to suggest that these women's childhoods have also been filled with severe and multiple losses (Bahr and Garrett, 1976; Cohen, 1988). Permanent relationships of a trusting nature are not the norm.

At the same time, homeless mentally ill women are survivors with many strengths. Their survival patterns and adaptive strategies, while on the streets, have been documented in the literature

(Manhattan Bowery Corporation, 1979; Martin, 1982; Hand, 1982). Their use of creative and nontraditional means of meeting basic needs and the cautious avoidance of others for purposes of self-protection point to strengths in adaptive capacity. It can be argued that physical survival on the streets for homeless mentally ill women would be impossible in the absence of considerable survival skills.

The women who participated in the Dinner Group all had histories of homelessness and all were diagnosed as mentally ill. They carried the traditional diagnoses of schizophrenia, bi-polar affective disorder, and a variety of personality disorders. Such diagnostic information, however, had limited value in predicting how the women would function within the group or in how each member would contribute to the character of the group as a whole. Furthermore, diagnostic formulations served to underscore the psychiatric disabilities of group members and raise questions in the workers' minds as to the ability of members to handle the responsibilities entailed in group participations. A functional formulation which highlighted the womens' problems-in-living proved more useful (Germain and Gitterman, 1980; Libassi, 1988).

The women who participated in the Dinner Group embody many of the characteristics of the female homeless mentally ill population described above. Life on the streets, in public shelters, and in psychiatric institutions had depleted many of their internal and external resources. Many of their daily living skills had atrophied over the years. Social supports such as family and friends were almost non-existent. Their sense of unpredictability in the environment and in their interpersonal relationships was considerable.

The women's ability to control the world around them had been systematically eroded. They were subject to starvation, exposure, arrest, and random acts of violence while living on the street. In institutions their lives were controlled by doctors, nurses, social workers, attendants, and guards. While survival on the streets required self-reliance, creativity, and independence, survival in institutions required submission to authority, conformity, and dependence. Pervading both experiences was the feeling of helplessness in the face of powerful external forces.

Though greater control over and predictability in the environment and in interpersonal relationships was possible once these women were housed, it was difficult for the women to perceive these possibilities. Many lived as if they were still on the street, reluctant to trust others and unable to feel safe. The fear of becoming homeless again made it difficult to abandon the adaptive techniques necessary for street life and mitigated against the formation of interpersonal relationships. The mistrust of mental health professionals and others who promised to "do good" (Gaylin et al., 1981) was pervasive. The perception of self as helpless in relationship to the physical and social environment was not easily unlearned. Thus, there were considerable obstacles to the development of interpersonal and daily living skills and to the empowerment of these women in relation to their environment.

## AGENCY CONTEXT

Our setting is an SRO hotel operated under the auspices of a nonprofit social agency. The hotel is staffed by paraprofessionals, 24 hours a day, 7 days a week. In this respect, the hotel is not a typical SRO, but rather is more similar to a group home or supportive residence. However, the agency operating the hotel is not part of, or funded by, the mental health system. The paraprofessional staff received no mental health training. Although most of the tenants are classified as mentally ill, psychiatric disability is not a criteria for tenancy. There was also no requirement that tenants accept or be involved with mental health services.

The status of the residence is further complicated by the presence of an on-site Community Support Systems (CSS) mental health program which operated in the hotel, 8 hours a day, 5 days a week. This program, nearly five years in operation, is affiliated with a graduate school of social work and serves as a field training site for student interns. The program is staffed by a social work supervisor, two paraprofessional case managers and two social work students.

As might have been expected, the CSS team was viewed with suspicion by many hotel residents at the time of the program's inception. The stigma attached to mental illness in this community was considerable. Few of the women admitted to having psychiatric hospitalizations and only 2 out of 36 were receiving psychiatric services. They were neither consulted about nor prepared for having a mental health program in their home. Such a beginning only served to compound the already existent mistrust of mental health professionals. Many of the women had been scarred by the harsh effects of prolonged institutionalization, the struggle for survival in the streets, and disappointing relationships with "helpers." Outsiders were not welcome, and posed a threat to the equilibrium in the hotel. While that state of being might have been less than ideal, it was at least known and consistent. Uncertainty was a threat unto itself. On the face of it, a mental health team was not welcome.

From the inception of the program there appeared to be a clash in values between the CSS team and the residents. The team emphasized the residents' right to receive services; the women asserted their right to refuse. The team believed themselves to be able to judge the women's need for service; the women believed themselves to know better. The team viewed mutual aid as critical to collective life; the women saw independence and individual prowess as key to survival. Interdependence was a threat.

The team's beliefs were fueled by their observations of what appeared to be overwhelming need, as well as their belief that they could create a sensitive and helpful relationship with the women. The tenants' beliefs were fueled by their prior disappointing experiences and their sense that they had no reason to expect that these professionals would be different from others. Caution and curiosity prevailed on both sides.

In the face of mutual reserve, the CSS team proceeded with its overall goal of rehabilitation and empowerment (Freire, 1970; Rose and Black, 1985). Objectives included maximizing opportunities through which the women could develop greater independence in daily living skills, develop increased interpersonal and social skills, and gain increased potency in relation to the environment. Linking the women to medical, psychiatric, and social services, was viewed as integral to meeting these objectives. Both individual and group services were developed to achieve these goals.

## THE GROUP SERVICE

The development of group services was a natural outgrowth of the women's lives together within the hotel. Residential settings have traditionally been fertile sites for the development of group services. People living together have a high degree of shared needs and a considerable potential for mutual aid (Forman, 1971). The high degree of isolation and limited social skills of these women, supported the belief that mutual aid within groups would be particularly helpful (Lee and Swenson, 1986; Shulman, 1985/86). Nonetheless, there were enormous obstacles to overcome if mutual aid was to flourish. Two residents describe the social environment in the hotel at the time of the program's inception:

> It was a madhouse, literally. The women were always bickering, arguing, fighting, and acting crazy . . . it was pretty depressing and people got on each other's nerves because they didn't have enough to do.

> It was deserted most of the time, we were cast out, isolated. There were just thirty-six women and we didn't have much to do with each other. There was nothing to do so people just stayed in their rooms. We didn't talk to each other. The women were idle, they argued and wanted to fight all the time. We had no unity, most of us knew each other before we lived here, from the shelter or from the street, but we did not have much to do with each other here. (Cohen, 1988)

The creation of activities through which social relationships could develop was the charge of the team. It was hoped that the group service program would engender mutual aid, strengthen daily living skills, provide opportunities for the enjoyment of leisure time, and promote a sense of self-mastery and effectiveness in relation to the environment. Ultimately, the team hoped helplessness and alienation would decrease. The Dinner Group was one of the first groups to be developed.

## THE DINNER GROUP

The Dinner Group emerged from observable need. The agency operating the hotel served two meals daily. Residents fended for themselves for dinner, some going to soup kitchens, a few purchasing their food, and many going without an evening meal. This group was designed to allow residents the opportunity to do the work which needed to occur if there was to be an evening meal. Tasks included: collectively planning a menu, developing a shopping list, shopping, managing a budget, preparing the meal, eating together, and cleaning up afterwards.

On the face of it, the contract between the workers and members was a simple one. The members wanted to plan and execute an evening meal and the workers were there to help them do so. They shared the recognition that the women could not manage this activity on their own. Beneath this clear manifest purpose lay many unstated issues and apprehensions, on both sides. The CSS team's covert purpose was that the women would develop: increased social and daily living skills, increased mutual aid, an increased sense of community, and increased responsibility for themselves. In contrast, although some group members enjoyed deciding what to eat, and a few appreciated the social nature of the group, the shared goal of most members was getting one free meal a week. They were wary of hidden agendas, particularly those of a psychiatric and social work nature.

Both worker and member orientations to the group had internal contradictions. Group members wanted to be independent and self-sufficient yet viewed themselves as powerless, expecting the hotel staff and the team to do things for them, rather than with them. The team wanted to counter the infantilization fostered by the hotel staff, yet also viewed the clients as severely disabled and in need of a great deal of directive assistance in negotiating the environment, and the tasks of this group in particular.

### Group Development and Shared Decision Making

While an analysis of the Dinner Group points to many rich themes for discussion, none is so central to the development of the group as is the tension between workers and clients around shared decision making. The workers experienced a powerful pull between their desire to create a participatory membership experience and their belief that a highly directive approach was necessary. This dialectical tension between prescriptiveness and permissiveness, between assertion and passivity, between process and outcome, became the critical variable shaping the development of the group as a whole and the experience for individual members. The pull between doing for and doing with the members can be seen throughout the life of the group.

### Group Composition

Although the Dinner Group participants were homogeneous in terms of gender, histories of homelessness and psychiatric diagnoses, group composition was essentially heterogeneous. Participants ranged in age from 30-71 and represented different racial, ethnic and religious backgrounds including: Caucasian, Black, Puerto Rican, Mexican American, Native American, Italian American, Irish American and Protestants, Catholics and Jews. Educational backgrounds included those without high school diplomas as well as those with college and master's education. Socioeconomic backgrounds were diverse as well. Almost all group members had been born into intact families but most lost contact with at least one parent through death, abandonment, or divorce prior to 21 years.

### How the Group Began: The First Year

The Dinner Group spanned a period of five years. Its story is told from the vantage point of the students who were assigned each academic year.

As the group began, feelings of trepidation and excitement were shared by the members and workers. Members cooperated and readily organized themselves for task accomplishment. Tasks were chosen based upon interest and competence, as well as upon a desire to avoid working with a disliked member. The members accepted the worker's prohibition that they could not shop for personal items when shopping for the group.

By the second month, differences among members and between the workers and the members began to appear. The workers were concerned that some members were too controlling and all members would not be included. Members who lost control and interfered with the working of the group were asked to leave. When members refused to rotate chores the issue of fairness was raised in the group.

Occasionally the group talked about other issues in the members' lives.

After only four short months the women displayed increased competence in previously difficult areas. They were able to go through the store alone, shopping was accomplished easily, and they became willing to let go of individual preferences. While co-operation among the women increased, tension between the workers and the members increased. It became necessary to establish and enforce some rules. The first rules were that all who wished to attend the dinner must attend the planning session and members were not allowed to fight or argue. There were few overt comments about the workers establishing and enforcing rules. The final dinner session was pleasantly executed. At the end of this first year the members were pleased with their individual progress and how the group had developed.

### The Group Continues: The Second Year

In the student worker's first log book entry, power struggles jumped off the page:

> Bella and Ruth started out taking over the group. We stopped them immediately and told them that we were leading the group. . . . A little while later Bella told me that I was mean because I told Mona that she could do something herself. . . . I didn't think I was being mean. I thought that was what the group was for, making the members more independent.

The workers found it necessary to make critical decisions for the group. Once Teresa arrived late and her task had been completed by another member. She refused to clean and left the group. When Bella insisted on making the spaghetti an hour early the workers had to take the spaghetti away. The members were told that the workers would have the final say over what goes on in the group. There were no immediate reactions from the members and the workers did not reach for any.

Tension over food and task assignments continued. Arguments came to physical blows. While the members were severely critical of each other, they hardly ever directly challenged the workers.

They did it indirectly as when Teresa broke a rule and gave out food to Lydia. The workers recognized that Teresa had felt sorry for Lydia because she was old and infirm. The workers did not feel comfortable to raise this conflict with the group. The members didn't push for this either.

By the third month the workers relinquished some authority to the group despite their concern about Bella and Connie who repeatedly tried to control things. The workers used intense persuasion to get the women to rotate chores in spite of Bella's reluctance.

The women became increasingly competent at welcoming and integrating new members. Challenges to the worker's authority increased subtly. The members complained, outside the group when Bella was barred from a session. The members had difficulty when Bella was not present. They said they needed her in the group. When Bella returned she was meek and mild. The workers still needed to decide which issues were open to group decision making and the group was able to carry them out. Only Bella and occasionally Connie differed with us.

Toward the end of the year Bella became upset over those who do not do enough and at the workers for protecting them. She became excessively angry and was asked to leave. For the first time another member supported Bella and directly disagreed with the workers. In the final group meeting the group ended on a high note. The members felt they had accomplished much and looked forward to the group starting again in the fall.

### A Small Shift Occurs: The Third Year

The members began the group by sharing the group's history. They emphasized task rotation and how the group was open to anyone who wanted to join. Everyone felt sad when Bella had a stroke and could not return to the group. The members wondered if they could manage without her. Some even suggested that they shouldn't continue because Bella was such an important part of the group. As the group proceeded, they saw that they could continue. Teresa moved into Bella's role and challenged "the rule" about rotating chores. The workers felt compelled to state that unless she took her turn with cooking, she could not participate in the group. She conceded.

The group appeared to be functioning well. Membership was stable and participants more often talked with each other and were willing to try new tasks. The workers felt that the members could manage their work with less intervention by the workers.

Rules continued to be used as the means of resolving differences and though they became fairly well defined within the group closeness among the members increased. Discussion about the death of Elaine's husband helped draw them together. As new members entered, it was the ongoing members who explained the group and said what they wanted it to be. The group was beginning to be more cohesive. New members were incorporated easily and all tasks handled well. Occasionally the workers spoke about the process of the group and continued to be less directive.

The members upheld the rule about no abusive behavior and no drinking. They even periodically commented on each others' behavior. Voting was still needed to make decisions. Members were receptive to majority rule but could make compromises. Individual members were stronger in presenting their points of view, others less dominating. The worker suggested that members shop without them because it was important for members to learn to manage on their own.

For the last meeting the workers decided to do all the chores. All the members had to do was eat and enjoy themselves. Workers and members shared closeness. They found it hard to believe that someone would give to them in this way.

### The Group as a Whole Is Stronger: The Fourth Year

The group began by the members informing the workers of the rules of the group. Though the process was not conflict free, tasks were handled well and easily.

It was unfortunate that damage from fire interrupted the Dinner Group for two months. The group resumed on a more collaborative note and at a high performance level. Everyone was happy when Tina ventured to the store herself for the first time.

Members began to make their own rules and for the first time spent an entire hour discussing conflict within the group. Members struggled with a rigid versus flexible application of rules. When members couldn't reach consensus the workers decided for them.

The members flexibly applying their rules was demonstrated by their allowing a disruptive member back into the group.

### The Group at Its Strongest: The Fifth Year

As the fifth year progressed old issues arose but appeared to be handled in new ways. For example, while structured voting was used to resolve differences, consensus decision making appeared more often. Frequently the workers posed issues to the group and suggested they decide how to resolve them. It became clear to the group and to the workers that only one worker was necessary and primarily on a consultative basis. The members were able to plan, shop and cook their meals without the worker's active assistance.

### CONCLUSION

This discussion of the Dinner Group is anchored in a practice strategy designed to enable members to become increasingly more powerful in relation to their interpersonal and environmental worlds. This practice orientation focuses upon the strengths of our homeless, mentally ill group members, rather than on their deficits. It emerges in an effort to counteract the effects of alienation, hopelessness, and despair, developed through life within psychiatric institutions and life on the streets. We are interested in a strong working group, a group mature in its development capable of satisfying members' needs. We expect that as member to authority and member to member relationships develop, so will the group as a whole (Berman-Rossi, 1987).

Most stage developmental literature suggests that in initial stages of group development members are primarily concerned with the power of the worker and must address this power relationship sufficiently so they can move on to develop intimacy with peers (Bennis and Shepard, 1956; Caple, 1978; Glassman and Kates 1983). Garland, Jones, and Kolodny (1973) add the dimension of power relationships among members as a vigorous component of the development of the group as a whole. Status, ranking, and role definitions, become important internal components of the working of the group as a whole. The development of the Dinner Group amply illustrates this literature.

The members' reconciling of the workers' power took place over the life of the group. Viewing the group over five years tells the story of how these women eventually became strengthened to assert their independence from the workers. Each year member to worker relationships, member to member relationships, and the group as a whole progressed. The yearly change of workers, and the open-ended nature of the group were significant elements influencing that rate of development (Shopler and Galinsky 1984).

The members' overall pleasure with the group, their instinctive cautiousness in relationships with peers and authorities and their fear of losing something valuable, inhibited them from more assert-ively dealing with the workers' power. Initially, the workers' fears that both they and the members were limited in their collective abil-ities to handle process issues inhibited the workers from opening up important matters to the group. Rules and formal voting became vehicles for establishing order and helping the group move to-gether. The eventual shift from the workers to a sharing of power was based on the recognition that not only were the members competent to handle group issues, but they were indeed theirs to handle. It was their group, just as the original workers had hoped it would be.

The workers' definition of function shifted from a "doing for" orientation to a "doing with" perspective, as they gained confi-dence in the women's abilities to handle issues in their lives. The cooking group provided a structure around which severely emotion-ally disabled women were able to sustain themselves and each other and to experience some new level of competence. These women were empowered through the group to better their lives and their surroundings.

## BIBLIOGRAPHY

Arce, A., Tadlock, M., Vergare, M., and Shapiro, S. "A Psychiatric Profile of Street People Admitted to an Emergency Shelter." *Hospital and Community Psychiatry*, Vol. 34, No. 9, 1983.
Bachrach, L. L. "The Homeless Mentally Ill and Mental Health Services: An Analytic Review of the Literature." In Lamb, R.H., editor, *The Homeless Mentally Ill: A Task Force Report of the American Psychiatric Association.* Washington, DC: The American Psychiatric Association, 1984.
Bachrach, L. L. "Chronic Mentally Ill Women: Emergence and Legitimation of

Program Issues." *Hospital and Community Psychiatry*, Vol. 36, No. 10, 1985.

Bahr, H. and Garrett, G. *Women Alone*. Lexington, MA: Lexington Books, 1976.

Baxter, E. and Hopper, K. *Private Lives/Public Spaces*. New York: Community Service Society, 1981.

Bennis, W. and Shephard, H. "A Theory of Group Development." *Human Relations*. 9(1956): 415-57.

Berman-Rossi, T. (1987). "Empowering Groups Through Understanding Stages of Group Development," Paper presented at the Ninth Annual Symposium on Social Work with Groups, Boston, MA.

Caple, R. "The Sequential Stages of Group Development." *Small Group Behavior*. 9:4(1978): 470-76.

Cohen, M. B. "Engaging the Homeless Mentally Ill." Unpublished paper, 1985.

Cohen, M. B. "Interaction and Mutual Influence in a Program for Homeless Mentally Ill Women." Unpublished PhD dissertation, The Florence Heller School for Advanced Studies in Social Welfare, Brandeis University, 1988.

Crystal, S. "Homeless Men and Homeless Women: The Gender Gap." *The Urban and Social Change Review*, Vol. 17, No. 2, 1984.

Forman, M. "The Alienated Resident and the Alienating Institution." *Social Work* 16, 2(1971): 47-54.

Freire, P. *Pedagogy of the Oppressed*. New York: Continuum Publishing Company, 1970.

Garland, J., Jones, H., and Kolodney, R. "A Model for Stages of Development in Social Work Groups." In Bernstein, S., editor. *Explorations in Group Work: Essays in Theory and Practice*. Boston: Milford House, Inc., 1973.

Gaylin, W. et al. *Doing Good: The Limits of Benevolence*. New York: Pantheon Books, 1981.

Germain, C. and Gitterman, A. *The Life Model of Social Work Practice*. New York: Columbia University Press, 1980.

Glassman, U. and Kates, L. "Authority Themes and Worker-Group Transactions: Additional Dimensions to the Stages of Group Development." *Social Work with Groups*. 6:2(1983): 33-52.

Golden, S. "Daddy's Good Girls: Homeless Women and Mental Illness." In Lefkowitz, R., and Withorn, A., editors, *For Crying Out Loud*. New York: Pilgrim Press, 1986.

Hand, J. "Shopping Bag Ladies of Manhattan." Unpublished PhD dissertation, The New School for Social Research, 1982.

Hopper, K. and Hamburg, J. *The Making of America's Homeless: From Skid Row to the New Poor, 1945–1984*. New York City: Community Service Society, 1984.

Lamb, R. H. "Deinstitutionalization and the Homeless" in Lamb, R. H., editor. *The Homeless Mentally Ill: A Task Force Report of the American Psychiatric Association*. Washington, DC: The American Psychiatric Association, 1984.

Lee, J. A. B. "No Place to Go: Homeless Women." In Gitterman, A. and

Shulman, L., editors, *Mutual Aid Groups and the Life Cycle*. Itasca, IL: F.E. Peacock Publishers, Inc., 1986.

Lee, J. and Swenson, C. "The Concept of Mutual Aid." In Gitterman, A. and Shulman, L., editors, *Mutual Aid Groups and the Life Cycle*. Itasca, IL: F.E. Peacock Publishers, Inc., 1986.

Levine, I. S. "Homelessness: Its Implications for Mental Health Policy and Practice." *Psychosocial Rehabilitation Journal*, Vol. 8, No. 1, 1984.

Levine, I. S. and Stockdill, J., "Mentally Ill and Homeless." In Jones, B., editor, *Treating The Homeless: Urban Psychiatry's Challenge*. Washington, DC: American Psychiatric Press Inc., 1986.

Libassi, M. F. "The Chronically Mentally Ill: A Practice Approach." *Social Casework*. 2:69(1988) 88-97.

Lipton, F. R., Sabatini, A., and Katz, S. E. "Down and Out in the City: The Homeless Mentally Ill." *Hospital and Community Psychiatry*, Vol. 34, No. 9, 1983.

Manhattan Bowery Corporation. *Shopping Bag Ladies: Homeless Women*. New York: Report to the Fund for the City of New York, April 1979.

Martin, M. A. "Strategies of Adaption: Coping Patterns of the Urban Transient Female." Unpublished PhD dissertation, Hunter College School of Social Work, 1982.

Morse, G. "Homeless People: A Typological Analysis and Gender Comparison." Unpublished PhD dissertation, University of Missouri, November 1984.

Putnam, J., Cohen, N., and Sullivan, A. "Innovative Outreach Services for the Homeless Mentally Ill." *International Journal of Mental Health*. Vol. 14, No. 4, 1986.

Rose, S. and Black, B. L. *Advocacy and Empowerment*. Boston: Routledge and Kegan Paul, 1985.

Rossi, P. H., Wright, J. D., Fisher, G. A., and Willis, G. "The Urban Homeless" Estimating Composition and Size." *Science*, Vol. 235, 1987.

Roth, D., Bean, J., and Johnson, E. *Homelessness in Ohio: A Study of People in Need*. Ohio: Department of Mental Health, Office of Program Evaluation and Research, 1985.

Schopler, J. and Galinsky, M. "Meeting Practice Needs: Conceptualizing the Open-Ended Group." *Social Work with Groups*. 7:2(1984):3-19.

Schwartz, W. "The Social Worker in the Group." The Social Welfare Forum. New York: Columbia University Press, 1961.

Shapiro, J. *Communities of the Alone*. New York: Association Press, 1971.

Shapiro, J. "Group Work with Urban Rejects in a Slum Hotel." In *The Practice of Group Work*. Schwartz, W. and Zalba, S., editors, New York: Columbia University Press, 1971.

Shulman, L. *The Skills of Helping Individuals and Groups*. Itasca, IL: F.E. Peacock Publishers, Inc., 1984.

Shulman, A.K. "Preface." In Rousseau, A.M., *Shopping Bag Ladies*. New York: Pilgrim Press, 1981.

Shulman, L. "The Dynamics of Mutual Aid." In Gitterman, A. and Shulman,

L., editors. ''The Legacy of William Schwartz: Group Practice as Shared Interaction.'' *Social Work with Groups*. 8:4(1985/86): 51-60.

Stoner, M. ''The Plight of Homeless Women.'' *Social Service Review*, Vol. 57, December, 1983.

United States Department of Health and Human Services. *Helping the Homeless: A Resource Guide*. Washington, DC: Department of Health and Human Services, 1984.

# Creating Community: Groupwork to Develop Social Support Networks with Homeless Mentally Ill

Marsha A. Martin
Susan A. Nayowith

**SUMMARY.** Group programs and the use of social group work skills can create social support networks and community among mentally ill homeless persons. Examples of groups developed by workers on a mobile mental health outreach unit on the streets, or a health/mental health team in a drop-in center and in a single room occupancy (SRO) hotel are presented. The programs demonstrate support of indoor living and effective maintenance of the homeless mentally ill persons in the community.

Homelessness, a major contemporary urban social problem has been studied in both formal and informal exploration of its many facets (Baxter and Hopper, 1981, 1982; Leaf and Cohen, 1982; Crystal, 1982; Hoffman, 1982; HUD, 1984; Brown et al., 1983; Bassuk, 1984; Crystal and Goldstein, 1984; Hopper and Hamburg,

Marsha A. Martin, DSW, is Assistant Professor at the Hunter College School of Social Work in New York City. She is a board member of the New York City Coalition of the Homeless, The New York City Coalition of Voluntary Mental Health, Mental Retardation, and Alcoholism Agencies, Inc., and Women in Need, Inc., a voluntary agency serving homeless women and their children. Susan A. Nayowith, MSW, is Program Supervisor at "Our Place," a day treatment program for homeless women sponsored by the Lenox Hill Neighborhood Association. She is formerly a social worker at the William F. Ryan Community Health Center Community Support Services Program servicing three SRO hotels on the upper westside of Manhattan.

79

1984; Roth et al., 1985; Struening et al., 1987). Causes of home-lessness have been identified and delineated: the absence and inade-quacy of low-cost housing, deinstitutionalization, hospitalization policies, unemployment, fragmentation of human services, chang-ing family structure, economic recession, increases in alcohol and substance use and abuse, and poverty. Exploration of the question "Who are the homeless?" has shown that they are men, women, children of all ages, all ethnic and racial origins, all educational and occupational levels, and all functional abilities. The extent of men-tal illness among the homeless has been variously estimated from 30 to 70% (Lee, 1986; Roth, 1986). Service needs have been identi-fied and assessed: shelter, food, clothing, services in shelters, alco-hol and substance abuse treatment, mental health treatment, medi-cal care, socialization, employment and vocational training, safety, permanent housing, case management services, and someone who cares (Martin, 1986; Lee, 1986). Much has been learned from these efforts to examine the problem, but little attention has been given to the social support systems among the homeless people and specifi-cally among the homeless mentally ill.

This paper discusses the development of social support networks, through the use of social group work, with the homeless mentally ill men and women in drop-in centers, shelters, and SRO hotels. Addi-tionally, the use of these networks to support "indoor living" is discussed using the experience of several programs serving the homeless in New York City.

The focus of attention in the 1960s on the impact of community on personal development paralleled the emerging literature on net-works. Joan Shapiro's discussion of "urban rejects" (1971) began to identify and make use of ways to understand and describe human interactions and the social work role within the context of an SRO hotel environment. Whether they developed naturally or were cre-ated for the purpose of support and problem-solving, personal and social support networks were found to exist and the nature of the life of the dispossessed in the community became more understand-able.

The discharge of mentally ill men and women from state psychi-atric centers to the community in the late 1970s through the deinsti-tutionalization policy resulted in large numbers of formerly domiciled state hospital patients moving into changing communities without the support of appropriate or adequate resources. Many of these former state hospital residents moved to the adult homes and SRO hotels, isolated from friends, family, and relationships of familiarity. Their psychosocial and housing needs quickly became evident and some social work attention turned to creating communities and social networks.

Prior to deinstitutionalization, assumptions about the needs of the chronic and seriously mentally ill individuals were based on a hospital/institutional model. Little attention had been given to the nature of the relationships of these individuals within the hospital, between themselves or with staff, nor to their readiness or ability to make successful adaptation to the community. Some individuals were returned to the hospital, some were placed in health related facilities, and some became homeless.

The mentally ill individuals who became homeless found it to mean more than being without a home. It meant being without the bonds which link individuals to a "network of interconnected social structures" (Caplow, 1965). For them, the state of homelessness involved being without the resources, internal as well as external, which are essential for meeting basic human needs. Homelessness meant being without a "set of linkages," without a "network."

Social networks have been defined as "the matrix of relationships that surround a person and the characteristics of those social ties" (Cohen, 1986; Mitchell, 1969). Further, they are "a specific set of linkages among a defined set of persons, with the additional property that the characteristics of these linkages as a whole may be needed to interpret the social behavior of the persons involved" (McIntyre, 1987; Mitchell, 1969). Abels and Abels speak about the absence of social networks: "Discontinuity in relationships weakens the capacity for collective personal integration of behavior. If individuals are unable to experience a sense of continuity of their own experiences within the context of other, structural occurrences of inequality, of alienation, and of isolation are spiralled" (1980, p. 32).

While public officials and private organizations struggle to identify remedies for the problem of inadequate housing and homelessness, rehabilitative efforts must acknowledge the adaptive process, including strengths and abilities of homeless mentally ill persons. Programming must be developed which facilitates the creation and re-creation of essential linkages/networks to support "indoor living."

The common belief concerning the homeless mentally ill assumes they are totally disaffiliated, withdrawn, passive, and unable to interact with others. However the programs in New York City which are described herein have found them to be eager participants in activities when their basic needs are addressed through the group. Utilizing the social group work method these programs have provided an array of supportive and rehabilitative services and facilitated the development of formal and informal social support networks among the residents of shelters, drop-in centers and SRO hotels.

The importance of the use of social group work in the development of social networks with the homeless mentally ill is underscored by Middleman and Goldberg's discussion of social work with groups:

> to qualify as social work with a group, the work of the practitioner must include attention to helping the group members gain a sense of each other and their groupness. . . . To qualify as "social" work with a group, the work of the practitioner must focus on helping the members develop a system of mutual aid. This occurs by encouraging communication among members. . . . The worker tries to enable the group to increase its autonomy so that it can continue as a self-help and mutual support group after the worker either withdraws completely or changes to the role of consultant or sponsor. . . . Just as the legitimate content of social work with groups can be therapy, legitimate content can also be skills training, understanding life themes, or managing life transitions. (Middleman and Goldberg, 1987)

The two programs which are described and discussed below grew out of state and city concerns for the homeless mentally ill living on the streets of two neighborhoods, New York City Midtown and Upper Westside. These two neighborhoods have experienced, during recent times, an urbanization process commonly described as "gentrification," a turning of low-cost housing stock into luxury and unaffordable housing. As a result large numbers of mentally ill persons, many of those who have been deinstitutionalized, are without housing and community supports. The Midtown Outreach Program (of the Manhattan Bowery Corporation or MBC) and the Community Support Systems Program (of the William F. Ryan Community Health Center) identify individuals at risk, assist in the location of stable, affordable housing and provide necessary and critical human services to "support indoor living" (Martin, 1982). Both programs have successfully utilized social group work methods with the goal of building community, mutual aid, and social networks.

## A MOBILE MENTAL HEALTH OUTREACH PROGRAM

The MBC Midtown Outreach Program, a mobile mental health outreach program, staffed with professional social workers, nurse practitioners, psychiatrists, physicians, and mental health aides, was designed to reach the chronically mentally ill men and women in the greater Times Square area of New York City. The persons served by the outreach program tend to fall into two categories: those with documentable histories of psychiatric intervention (both institutional and community-based) and those without such histories but still requiring mental health care and treatment in order to live independently in the community. A primary task was defined as creating access to the necessary systems of care.

All the work with the clients is performed in the community, often on the streets, in the bus and train stations, shelters and drop-in centers. Upon approach, team members assess the prospective client and may make suggestions about needs and resources. If the homeless person is not immediately interested in assistance, the team will offer a flyer which describes the program and includes a telephone number to call. Even though a person may refuse aid, the outreach teams will continue contacts and encourage the use of their services and alternatives to living in the street. Most of the clients with whom the team works are disaffiliated and severely ill.

The Midtown Outreach Program is divided into two components: the street teams and the medical/psychiatric outreach teams. The outreach teams approach men and women on the streets. The medical/psychiatric teams provide on-site clinic services in private voluntary shelters and drop-in centers. Both components use groups in their comprehensive service delivery model. The shower and newspaper groups will be discussed as examples of the building of community, mutual aid and social networks.

### The Shower Group

The shower group was formed by a street outreach team as an outcome of its weekly escorting of homeless men by a street outreach team to a drop-in center where they could shower, receive clean clothing and be seen by the medical/psychiatric team. The group members were Jim, a mildly retarded overweight white male in his late thirties, Philip, in his early sixties, a self-detoxified recovering alcoholic with alcohol hallucinosis, and Kevin, a young white paranoid schizophrenic suffering from feelings of persecution. Their initial contact with staff in the van formed the basis for developing relationships and interactions among themselves which in time carried over to relationships independent of the team workers. The men began to show concern for others by asking for individuals who were not at their usual pick-up spots at the specified time. Their concern for others served to remind them of the possibilities they faced themselves.

Over time when the opportunity arose for the three men to be placed in housing their connection with a structured task-centered program played a significant role in helping them to become oriented to the new environment. Jim, Philip, and Kevin were able to address issues among themselves about moving into a new residence at first in the van, and thereafter in the hotel. Issues developed around the men's ideas of living indoors. Jim's enthusiasm about the move did not assuage his concern about Philip. He worried that Philip would not keep his room clean enough to remain in the hotel and offered to help when needed. The ability of the two men to plan support for one another in the new environment demonstrated to the workers their capacity for relationship in supportive and concrete ways.

An important aspect of a worker's job begins when a room becomes vacant and available to them for a client. Questions to be answered are: What structure is provided in the hotel? Are there on-site workers who provide services including social services, food services, medical and/or psychiatric care? Does the landlord remain on the premises for the duration of the day? Is the superintendent available, and if so, when? Who else lives in the building? Does someone have the role of helping others when needed? And, will that person be interested in having a formal introduction to the new resident(s)? The worker placing a client needs to use her/his knowledge of the client and familiarity of the environment to provide a match and transition which encourages the attainment of positive growth on behalf of both the client and the environment.

Once Jim, Philip, and Kevin moved into the hotel they began actively helping one another. Jim and Philip moved in one month before Kevin. They shared in cooking and shopping. They reminded each other about appointments scheduled with the MBC workers. Each man was able to meet new residents independently to whom they then introduced each other. Initially they were very attached not only to one another but to the workers. Workers must understand they are an important part of the social network for the clients and they must use their relationship in a purposeful way, as they are seen both as a part of the support system and as role models.

When Kevin became a resident several weeks later, Jim and Philip shared with their new neighbors their excitement about Kevin's upcoming move. All the carefully planned and executed preparations paved the way for a smooth transition for Kevin. At the time of his arrival he was greeted as the "new guy, a friend of Jim and Philip." While he had to meet his own neighbors and become accustomed to living indoors he was supported by the group members, the MBC team, and the other hotel support persons who had come to know and like the first two residents. He could depend on the support of the others. Perhaps more importantly, he was encouraged by their ability to "make it" and therefore he felt optimistic that he had a chance himself.

### Drop-In Center Newspaper Group

At an MBC drop-in center for homeless women, considered the first step off the street, women came to sit in chairs throughout the day and night, receive food, clothing, and other social service support. The MBC medical/psychiatric team members noticed that several of the women discussed current events raised by newspaper articles or television shows. They decided to build on the informal grouping in order to develop a time limited formal group activity with a goal of introducing themselves and the services of the team to the women. The women were intrigued by the newspaper activity and the opportunity to talk together with workers about many topics of interest. Subsequently the members brought other homeless women for participation in the group as well as in the MBC health/mental health clinic program. The structure of the newspaper group facilitated easy interaction between the group members and the staff, strengthening the functioning of the medical/psychiatric team in the drop-in center. While in the past the women appeared to be withdrawn and isolated from each other, the newspaper group allowed each to participate according to her abilities and to experience a social role in what was becoming for them the rudiments of a support system.

## GROUPS IN SRO HOTELS

The Ryan Community Support Systems Program provides on-site medical and psychiatric care to deinstitutionalized formerly homeless chronically and seriously mentally ill men and women in three single room occupancy (SRO) hotels on Manhattan's Upper Westside. Using a team approach, which includes case management and rehabilitation services, the Ryan program attempts to meet the needs of hotel residents through on-site medical and psychiatric clinics, the daily dispensation of medication, assistance with activities of daily living (ADL) skills, concrete services, and group programs in the area of recreation, socialization, education and support.

### The Bingo Group

Group work was a basic part of the plan by which to develop community and natural network systems among residents in the SRO hotels. Through groups the range of the resident's needs and abilities could be addressed. The staff assessed the need for socialization, rehabilitation, and psychiatric care for many residents who had not been involved in the organized activity offered. To this end, a weekly Bingo group was formed. It consisted of at least ten residents, seven of whom participated for at least three years.

Initially the preparation for the Bingo group activity was carried by the worker in order to provide structural support for the members (Kurland, 1982). Early on the worker asked or reminded potentially interested participants to attend. The hotel management also helped by reminding members to look for other tenants who seemed to enjoy participating. In time the members began to demonstrate the capacity for concern about others by looking out for one another. Residents in the hotel began to greet one another by saying, "Are you going to the game?" "What time will it be held?" "Do they need any help?"

There were three categories of participants. First there were persons involved on a daily basis with each other to meet their ADL needs. Then there were the residents who adapted to the structure initiated by the groups but retreated to their rooms when no group or clinic or formal activity was in process. Finally there were the persons who attended the group because they were sitting in the living room at the time it was being held but whose functioning was limited to concrete exchanges. Most participants had histories of extended or regular psychiatric hospitalizations for some variation of schizophrenia as defined in the DSMIII.

In an effort to draw on and develop strengths, residents were encouraged to attend for any reason, whether they were in need of extra food, toiletries, companionship or advice. One woman recommended the group to her neighbor, a person who was regularly asking for canned food: "The Bingo group is a place where you can get free food and even if you do not win you'll get a prize." The worker encouraged participants to reach out to isolated people with limited networks to join the group as a way to meet others.

Slowly as a core group of members developed, so also roles with group expectations attached to the function emerged. The members found they would depend on certain persons to call the numbers, set up the prizes, distribute the snack, and help to clean up. Within the preparation, play, and ending structure of the game there was opportunity for the members to experience a beginning level of mutuality with one another and the worker, carrying these relationships over into the daily life of the SRO Hotel. Persons who were connected with one another began to verbalize their concerns for each other. Residents who stayed in their rooms except when there was a structured program began spending time together in the living room. Residents who showed the most limited functioning began to ask other tenants to help them meet their primary needs as well as to share ideas and small talk with them. Clients became related to the worker. They were invested in how much rest she needed to be able to stay in the position or how well she was eating!

The Bingo game begins when the residents are seated around the parameter of the social service living room. A card table is set up with prizes and the number caller equipment. The worker assumes the tasks of getting the members to the activity on time, buying the agreed upon goods for prizes, providing the snacks, and by playing two Bingo cards. She facilitates verbal interaction before, during and after the actual game using the skill of observation throughout the game in order to foster network building. Who sits where? Who says what to whom? Who demonstrates support to whom? Dyads and triads become important indicators of relationships which exist or are growing among group members or residents. The Bingo group is an open group even though there are ten to twelve regular members who conduct the activity. Not having a door allows tenants to stop by and visit the residents who are playing Bingo. As the activity proceeds over time the worker can identify existing networks. The worker teaches about, encourages, and strengthens the formation and further development of social networks and the building of community within the SRO.

> Once the group begins to trickle in members begin to volunteer to help with setting up the game supplies. Ms. L, as usual, is keeping the room clean before and after the game. The three regular group members assist the worker in putting out the prizes, snacks, and extra chairs. The regular number caller, who comes down following a room visit from the worker earlier in the morning and a buzz from the front desk, enters and prepares her area for work.
>
> The group today is comprised of ten female senior citizens,

two male seniors, two men in their thirties, one Spanish speaking middle-aged man, and two people in their twenties. The worker begins greeting the members as they are seated or arrive and encourages conversation among players. She asks, How are you today? Did you get your paper filled out at the center? Have you asked the other tenants if they had a similar situation and then what course did they pursue and recommend? Today individuals seem to be asking one another without prompting from the worker for information and advice. When Ms. Q is ready to begin calling the game begins.

Ms. B takes a can of vanilla pudding, as she does each time she wins. Ms. B is not the only group member to take the same prize for each winning. Everyone does and as usual members know well who likes which gift. Last week the store did not have the standard fare and since the gifts were different there was an observable pall over the game. That is not true today. There are two winners for each game. Ms. B as usual wins a second game. She has difficulty remembering that each player may only win one time per game. The game proceeds and most players stay for the full period of time. Some leave as their neighbors or friends come by to speak with them.

The end of the game period developed special meaning for the group. Here they caught up on news from one another. As the clean-up process continued they exchanged ideas and information. Hotel events were discussed. Recently one member was worried because the electricity in her room was out for the day. Another member invited her to stay in her room until the problem was solved. The members were concerned about a tenant who had fallen out of her chair earlier in the week and was hospitalized. The worker brought them information about the ill woman's status.

In another example Ms. S became agitated when her neighbor was evicted. Some time ago Ms. S had been harassed by a man who is currently in jail. Now the empty room across the hall, the violence with which the tenant had left, and the unresolved concern and real fears about living in an SRO hotel environment were creating excess anxiety for her. The Bingo group members were able to offer their assistance and support by visiting with Ms. S in her room, attempting to work out a system whereby she might feel safe and regularly checking in on her.

Ms. F was an elderly woman who became hospitalized after undressing on Broadway. She was stabilized on prolixin and discharged from a local hospital. Immediately following her hospital leave she required attention to enable her to cope with her environment and to care for herself. Two women hotel receptionists helped Ms. F with dressing, eating, money management, and reminders to take her medication. She became identified with the group worker and became a regular participant in the Bingo group. She came for both concrete services and support. The group members were surprised at her ability to play Bingo and yet were positive in telling her how well she was doing. The members continued to look out for Ms. F and she would go to members when she had needs to be met, demonstrating some level of ability to interact with others. On a regular basis, Ms. F took on the job of reporting who had been waiting for the worker and what the person wanted. Her role in the structure of the hotel social network became integrated to provide a service for herself and others.

### The Cooking Group

The cooking group demonstrated how residents continued carrying on roles they learned in the group even after its dissolution. The basic group was comprised of five residents, four females and one male. Two women regularly prepared salad. Their task was considered special to them and they rarely accepted a change of menu. The hot meal preparers took pleasure in knowing how to cook. They also had a set formula for making specific dishes and any minor fluctuation created stress.

Throughout the group period residents regularly came to check on the food. Talk about preparation and serving kept everyone busy. A system of payment for the food was instituted for those who did not participate in the cooking, but wished to eat the meal. "Jobs" included participation in a delivery service. Clients could be involved by taking lunches to homebound residents and then reporting on their status and potential needs to the group members. This carried over into the weekend and holiday periods. They knew how to get emergency help if needed. Extra food was distributed to needy individuals in the hotel. Members offered to cook meals for one another when stoves were not functioning.

When the group was formally terminated one member continued to make lunch on Friday, cooking day. The woman became known by others as a person who cooked for her friends but who also took care of some of the more decompensated psychiatric individuals in the building. Ms. E was able to use the skills restored to her in the group experience to become a major food provider in the hotel. Her role in the hotel helped to build her self-esteem, seemed to have an effect on the number of times she herself decompensated, and enriched the community life in the hotel.

## CONCLUSION

In summary, the use of group work methodology provides the social worker with the professional tools by which to promote the development of social networks. These can maintain mentally ill homeless persons both while they are living on the streets and in the transition to "indoor" living. Group work methods which place emphasis on outreach to members, provision of structured supportive activity, and linkage to medical/psychiatric and entitlement resources enable the workers to create communities in environments prone to disorganization and disaffiliation.

The worker interacts with these painfully distressed people, conscious of being the mediator in the social network, acting as support, resource, linkage, and facilitator. Through the use of social groupwork skill, the social worker becomes a part of ongoing life processes with a critical role in the creating of community.

## REFERENCES

Abels, S.L. and Abels, P. "Social Group Work's Contextual Purposes." *Social Work with Groups*. Vol. 3, No. 3, Fall 1980.

Bassuk, E. "The Homeless Problem." *Scientific America* 25(1), 1984.

Baxter, E. and Hopper, K. "The New Mendicancy: Homeless in New York City." *American Journal of Orthopsychiatry*, 52, 1982.

Baxter, E. and Hopper, K. *Private Lives/Public Spaces: Homeless Adults on the Streets of New York City*. New York: Community Service Society, 1981.

Brown, C. et al. "The Homeless of Phoenix: Who Are They? And What Do They Want?" Phoenix, Arizona. Phoenix South Community Mental Health Center, 1983.

Caplow, T. et al. "Homeless." *International Encyclopedia of the Social Sciences*. New York: MacMillan, 1968.

Cohen, C. and Adler, A. "Assessing the Role of Social Network Interventions with an Inner-City Population." *American Journal of Orthopsychiatry*, 56 (2) 1986.

Collins, A. and Pancoast, D. *Natural Helping Networks: A Strategy for Prevention*. Washington, DC. National Association of Social Workers, 1976.

Compton, B. and Galaway, B. *Social Work Processes*. Homewood, Illinois: The Dorsey Press, 1984.

Crystal, S. *Characteristics of First Time Users of New York City Shelters*. New York, New York: Human Resources Administration, 1982.

Crystal, S. and Goldstein, M. *The Homeless in New York City Shelters*. New York, New York: Human Resources Administration, 1982.

Gartner, A. and Reisman, E. (eds.) *The Self-Help Revolution*. New York, New York: Human Sciences Press, 1984.

Hoffman, S. et al. "Who Are The Homeless?" Report of New York State Office of Mental Health. New York, New York, 1982.

Hopper, K. and Hamburg, J. *The Making of America's Homeless from Skid Row to New Poor*. New York, New York: Community Services Society, 1984.

Kurland, R. *Group Formation: A Guide to the Development of Successful Groups*. Monograph. Albany, New York: SUNY School of Social Welfare, 1982.

Leaf, A. and Cohen, M. *Providing Services for the Homeless: The New York City Program*, New York, New York: Human Resources Administration, 1982.

Lee, J. "No Place to Go: Homeless Women." In *Mutual Aid Groups and the Life Cycle*. Edited by Gitterman, A. and Schulman, L. Illinois: The Peacock Press, 1986.

Maguire, L. "The Interface of Social Workers with Personal Networks." *Social Work with Groups*. Vol. 3, No. 5, 1980.

Martin, M.A. *The Implications of NIMH Supported Research for Homeless Mentally Ill Racial and Ethnic Minority Persons*. Rockville, Maryland: National Institute of Mental Health, 1986.

Martin, M.A. "Strategies of Adaption: Coping Patterns of Urban Transient Females." Unpublished dissertation. Columbia University, 1982.

McIntyre, E.C.G. "Social Networks: Potential for Practice." *Social Work*. Vol. 36, No. 6, 1986.

Middleman, R.R. and Goldberg, G. "Social Work Practice With Groups," in *Encyclopedia of Social Work*. Silver Springs, Maryland: National Association of Social Workers, 1987.

Mitchell, J. "Concept and Use of Social Networks," in *Social Networks in Urban Situations*. J. Mitchell (ed.), Manchester, England: Manchester University Press, 1969.

Roth, D. et al. *Homelessness in Ohio*. Columbia, Ohio: Ohio Department of Mental Health, 1985.

Shapiro, J. "Group Work in a Slum Hotel," in *The Practice of Group Work*. Schwartz, Wm. and Zalba, S. (eds.), New York, New York: Columbia University Press, 1971.

Swenson, C. "Social Networks, Mutual Aid, and the Life Model of Practice," in *Social Work Practice: People and Environments*. Germain, C. (ed.), New York: Columbia University Press, 1979.

Struening et al. *Characteristics of Residents of New York City Shelter System*. New York, New York: New York State Psychiatric Institute, 1987.

U.S. Department of Housing and Urban Development. *A Report to the Secretary on the Homeless and Emergency Shelters*, Washington, DC: U.S. Government Printing Office, 1984.

# Social Group Work in a Soup Kitchen: Mobilizing the Strengths of the Guests

Irene Glasser
Jane Suroviak

**SUMMARY.** The soup kitchen functions as a symbolic living room for people whose marginality takes the forms of low income, long term unemployment, debilitating physical conditions, serious mental illness, loneliness, and separation from conventional family relationships. Through use of group work, indigenous leadership in the social network of the soup kitchen was strengthened to foster self-help—people helping each other.

Soup kitchens have become pervasive as community groups respond to the homeless and hungry who are visible throughout the metropolitan areas. The well functioning soup kitchen offers its guests several hours of warmth, nourishment, sociability and acceptance. It is able to provide asylum in the original meaning of "a place of sanctuary." The guests form an amalgam of people out of the mainstream of life who are at times referred to as "street people" (Bachrach 1984), in recognition of all of the time they spend on the streets and in other public places.

For many of the guests, the soup kitchen becomes the very center of their social existence. The soup kitchen may be seen as a particular adaptation to contemporary North American life, serving as a niche for a segment of the poor who are considered "marginal" to

---

Irene Glasser, MSW, PhD, is affiliated with Eastern Connecticut State University, Willimantic, CT. Jane Suroviak, MS, is the former Director of Covenant Soup Kitchen, Willimantic, CT.

the dominant culture. This marginality takes the forms of low income, long term unemployment, debilitating physical conditions, serious mental illness, loneliness, and a separation from conventional family relationships. Because of these conditions, most soup kitchen guests lack the sources of human contact that people take for granted in work, family relationships and consumer activities. The soup kitchen functions as a symbolic living room for this segment of people in poverty, in a manner reminiscent of "Tally's Corner" for a group of urban men in Washington D.C. (Liebow, 1967) and the tavern for alcoholic men (Dumont, 1967).

Today's soup kitchens differ from most health and social service agencies in ways that make them especially appealing to some of the poorest and most disaffiliated members of contemporary society. No records, folders, charts or other accoutrements of the modern agency are kept. People who come to the soup kitchen are termed guests or diners by the soup kitchen staff, instead of the clients, patients or recipients of other programs. The term guest also has a quasi-religious connotation in that soup kitchen staff who often have a religious motivation for their work see the guest or stranger who sits down to eat as being the embodiment of God (Rendle, 1984).

Our work in the Tabernacle Soup Kitchen* in a small, former industrial center in the Northeast, has enabled us to discover a variety of strategies for building on the strengths of the guests who eat in the dining room daily. The soup kitchen provided us with an opportunity to test out several ideas in the tradition of social group work. We were interested in how we could help the soup kitchen support and sustain the power of mutual aid within the dining room. The examples presented here come from the Community Resources Courses and the Food Clubs which have been conducted in the Tabernacle Soup Kitchen.

The methodology for our work comes out of our backgrounds in social work, anthropology and the ministry. Our work includes five years of ethnographic study and of doing social work (Glasser) and four years of being the director of the soup kitchen (Suroviak). The ethnography is fully described in the book *More Than Bread: Eth-*

---

*The name Tabernacle Soup Kitchen, and all the other names in this paper are pseudonyms.

*nography of a Soup Kitchen* (Glasser, 1988). In it, anthropological methods are utilized in order to discover what about the setting makes it so appealing to so many of the guests who are disaffected with other services. The anthropological methods of waiting and watching, of recording extensive field notes, and of some linguistic analyses helps us understand the setting from an insider's, or *emic* point of view. The cultural themes of the soup kitchen were found to be sociability, acceptance and affiliation, which create an ambiance in which mutual aid can potentially flourish.

## SELF-HELP IN THE SOUP KITCHEN

Throughout the world, there are examples of health care and other human services programs in which local people are trained to deliver services to their own people. This model is a way of bridging the cultural gap that often exists between the professional world and the world of the consumer of health or human services. At times, the indigenous worker is seen as the *only* way to reach underserved populations in a culturally congruent manner. Central to the idea of the indigenous worker is the identification of individuals who have demonstrated leadership potential or who are central figures within their social network and are willing to become involved with others to share their knowledge.

The soup kitchen provided us with an excellent opportunity to reach and engage people who are most often labelled as "unmotivated" for traditional sources of help. We discovered that, as Margot Breton (1985) has discussed, if we started with an understanding of what people were motivated to do, helped them discover their own competence, created optimal challenges, and utilized the naturally forming support networks, we would be successful in reaching a large number of the guests.

## COMMUNITY RESOURCES COURSES

After becoming aware of the general sociability, acceptance and affiliation of the setting, we wanted to see if these attributes could be in any way enhanced through a social group work project with some of the guests. For example, if some of the guests affiliated with each other in social networks, could the degree of support within the network be increased? Could the advice people often give each other about resources in the community be based on more accurate information? Could the atmosphere of sociability and acceptance be enlarged to include some of the guests who are "loners"? Would a group of guests come to regularly scheduled classes, or would the continual life crises that we knew existed for most of the guests interfere? Could classes be designed so as not to be perceived as too structured and alien to the nonthreatening ambiance of the soup kitchen?

In order to address some of these issues, we conducted three projects in self-help within the soup kitchen in the form of Community Resources Courses in the spring of 1984, in the fall of 1985, and in the winter of 1987. A total of twenty-one guests completed the course, with two guests taking it twice and one guest taking it three times. Each course consisted of approximately twelve hours of instruction, in twice weekly sessions. We searched for guests whom others looked to for support and guidance, and invited these guests to join the course. Several guests indicated their interest in the course and were invited to come. In addition, several noontime announcements were made about the classes to the entire dining room, in order to avoid excluding any guests who wanted to come.

Ideally the participants in the training course would be members of a social support network, and should have some of the traditionally defined leadership qualities, such as the "capacity to stimulate the group, mobilize activities, synthesize thinking . . ." (Hartford, 1971) or be, in the words of the Inuit, "the one to whom all listen" (Nanda 1984). However, not every guest who had some of these characteristics was interested in or able to participate in the training.

Peggy, for example, was a dominant person within a social network of soup kitchen regulars who were middle-aged women. She had the respect of many of the guests, who looked up to her as she gave out information about welfare programs (at times inaccurately) and passed judgment on the other guests by her comments and facial expressions. Though often approached, Peggy was not interested in the classes. She did, however, say that two people at her table were interested, and one became an active participant.

Most of the classes were held in the large room above the dining room of the soup kitchen, except for three sessions during which the class visited community agencies. Babysitting was provided through funds from a local foundation, in order to enable people with children to attend. The grant money also paid for notebooks, pens, graduation certificates, and graduation presents of a cardboard-file carrying-case for the numerous brochures and papers accumulated by the class participants.

The first course was given bilingually in English and in Spanish for the Spanish speaker in the course. This was moderately successful in that he felt more included and received most of the information. Most of the time the other class members were patient during the interpreting periods.

## The Members/Students

The following is a brief description of the six soup kitchen guests who successfully completed the first course.

Marie was a woman in her forties of Portuguese descent, who came to the soup kitchen daily with her three daughters and her five grandchildren. She lived in an apartment on Main Street, and had custody of Steve, her five-year-old grandson. Marie was the focal person of a social network that included her daughters, their children, and their friends.

Esther was a white woman in her fifties who was disabled by arthritis and lived in a low-income housing project. She was a soup kitchen regular who sat at Peggy's table. Like many of the other women at the soup kitchen, she had children who were in and out of trouble with the law. She was well respected by the other, older women of the soup kitchen.

Alan was a young white man in his twenties who spent most of his mornings at the soup kitchen, in addition to working at a maintenance job on the second shift. He had lived in Middle City all of his life, and had held various low-skilled jobs for short periods as well as being sporadically unemployed. Alan was a member of a group of young men and women in the soup kitchen. He was also involved in a fundamentalist Protestant church that attracted some of the young soup kitchen guests.

Pedro was a Puerto Rican man in his fifties who was a workfare kitchen worker and a guest in the soup kitchen. He lived at the Hotel Paradise, the local welfare hotel, and was a part of the group of men who stood in front of the hotel for many hours each day. He was a warm, congenial man, who, despite his limited English ability, was a friend to many of the soup kitchen guests.

Jane was a white woman in her fifties who had a motor impairment which made her speech and gait awkward. She lived in a low-income housing project and worked at a sheltered workshop before coming to the soup kitchen each day. Although Jane did not appear to be a regular member of any particular group in the soup kitchen, she was on friendly terms with everyone. Jane had taken in a homeless young woman during the previous fall, and in spite of numerous problems in trying to get the woman to leave, obviously enjoyed her role and status as a helping person.

Barbara was a heavily tattooed white woman in her twenties, who had recently moved to Middle City. Her marriage had recently broken up and she had given birth to a baby who died shortly thereafter. She was a workfare kitchen worker and guest at the soup kitchen, and lived at the Hotel Paradise. She was a very friendly, popular young woman, friends with almost all of the soup kitchen guests. Barbara was one of the most active class participants and eventually became a spokesperson for the soup kitchen community as a whole.

In addition to the guests described, there was Sue, a soup kitchen "regular" who came to half of the classes, but referred to herself as a "visitor" to the class rather than a class participant. Sue was a young woman who was recovering from an almost fatal mugging and subsequent coma. She was interested in joining the group, but made it clear that she could not make a commitment to attend all of the classes. She told me that she could not visualize herself as being of any help to anyone else since she could barely keep track of her own life. Sue was, in fact, a very lively class participant when she did attend, and though not a leader within the soup kitchen, she was in fact embedded in a social network of other young women who lived with her at the Hotel Paradise.

### The Class/Group Structure

Professionals in the community were invited to present materials to the class on each topic. Most of the professionals were enthusiastic about the idea of the indigenous worker concept as applied to a soup kitchen, and they treated the participants in the class with respect. The participants appeared to be able to absorb much of the information provided by the community professionals. The social worker from an anti-poverty agency discussed legal rights in applying for town welfare, an issue faced by many of the soup kitchen guests because town assistance workers had been known to harass potential recipients in order to discourage them from applying for welfare. The housing expert discussed the increasing shortage of low-income apartments. Out of the discussion (as well as other efforts) came a program that has gathered funds to be used to guarantee the security deposits for people on town welfare who would otherwise not be able to move out of their rooms at the single-room-occupancy hotel and boarding houses. One of the class participants, Barbara, became the soup kitchen community representative to the group of professionals involved with this housing effort.

Another highlight of the classes was the talk given by a drug and alcohol counselor who was a former heroin addict. All the participants were experienced, or were close to someone who was experienced in drug and alcohol use. They were particularly interested in drug combinations and their cumulative effect. The class was also invited to tour the local therapeutic community which none of the class members had ever entered before.

During one of the sessions, a community nutritionist brought snacks for the group, which were examples of nutritious, economical foods. She also brought empty boxes of common products, in order to demonstrate the art of reading the ingredients list. In addition she brought a seven-foot-tall mannequin, with detachable internal organs, in order to demonstrate digestive processes. The class was lively and the participants were open-minded about trying the somewhat unorthodox foods suggested by the nutritionist.

## The Class/Group Mediates

The most confrontive class took place at the local mental health clinic and illustrated the mediating function of both the group worker and the group (Shulman and Gitterman, 1986). We met at the clinic with four members of the treatment staff, in order to learn about the treatment modalities offered by the clinic. As the informational session began, Jane broke into a tirade of tears and anger, stating how little the clinic had helped her when she was caring for her dying mother who was engaging in bizarre behaviors. The director of services said that the clinic does not usually make home visits, except for the Hispanic unit. This reply made Jane even angrier. Sue talked about her dislike of the clinic's psychiatric halfway house, and how she had purposely broken all of the rules so that she would be thrown out. At the end of the session, Marie, who had been uncharacteristically quiet for the full session, stated that the clinic had done nothing for her and her fourteen-year-old daughter who was truant from school, and whom the courts were threatening to send to a reform school. To this, the clinic spokesperson said that the clinic was best able to handle mental health problems and not social problems! At the end of the class, the group members waited for Marie as she went to find the counselor in charge of her daughter's case, in order to confront her. It was during this session that the potential power of a group of service consumers became evident. The guests, usually treated as passive clients of the mental health clinic, had become empowered to confront the professionals. It is difficult to assess the impact of Marie's confrontation, but her daughter was eventually sent to a group home which is often considered (by mental health professionals) a better alternative than remaining on the streets or going to reform school. Throughout the rather emotional session, the worker offered support for the class to confront the "experts."

### Graduation

At the completion of the training course, a graduation ceremony was held during the noon hour at the soup kitchen, in front of some hundred or so guests. A list of the names of the six guests who completed the training was then posted in a prominent place near the coffee pot, and the director of the soup kitchen made public reference to the graduates of the program for several weeks after the end of the training program, suggesting them as a resource for people with problems in the areas of the trainee's studies.

## Follow Up

In order to assess the impact the indigenous workers might have had on the other soup kitchen guests, two follow-up sessions were held. During the first session, two weeks after the end of the program, Alan, Marie, Barbara, and Esther said that they had been approached by guests who wanted to know more about employment and housing programs. During this session, we also discussed the situation of a guest who was acting in a rather bizarre manner in the dining room, walking about aimlessly, carrying an old rock magazine wherever she went, and spending inexplicably long periods of time in the ladies' room. The response from the group was that they wanted to stay far away from this guest, so that she would not "hit" them.

This example pointed up a major complication of guests becoming involved with people outside their usual social networks. If one of the class members did become involved with this disturbed guest, it would be impossible to end the relationship at one o'clock in the afternoon, when the soup kitchen was over. The class participants were all members of the low-income communities and would not be able to "turn off" their contacts at five o'clock the way middle-class professionals do.

Immediately after the training ended, Marie entered a job-training program, and has been employed ever since at an egg farm. Barbara continued to work at the soup kitchen for six months after the course. During that time she moved out of the hotel and into an apartment. While still on workfare, she joined a training course for kitchen workers held at the soup kitchen and graduated from it. She was then hired at a local fast-food restaurant and was still working there over a year later. She was being trained for a management position. She also spoke in public on the needs of the guests in regards to housing. Alan continued to work at various jobs and began to talk about applying to college. He became a leader of a local tenants' rights organization and was involved in helping conduct a local politician's campaign. Alan recently brought a teenager to a youth service agency, telling the counselor there that he had learned of the agency from the Community Resources Course of two years before.

The two guests who returned to work point to an important difference between the indigenous worker in more traditional cultures in which the idea has been tried, and the indigenous worker idea in the soup kitchen. In other cultures, successful workers are expected to remain within the culture, at least for a period of time. On the other hand, "success" in terms of the soup kitchen culture often means finding employment and then leaving the soup kitchen.

Two further community counseling courses were held at the soup kitchen. Each time the course was refined so that it was more congruent with the guests. For example, a shorter class format that ended well before the meal was implemented. During the second course a central figure within the group of young mothers joined. By the third course at least some of the "recruiting" was accomplished by the guests who had been involved with the previous courses. The topics covered included welfare, alcohol and drug rehabilitation services, health, mental health, employment, education, rape crisis, and battered women's services. In addition, the supervisor of the local protective service agency came to discuss child abuse and neglect with the class. Many of the members of the class had had direct contact with protective services, by having been reported (or "turned in" in the soup kitchen vernacular) for being suspected of abuse or neglect of their children. Despite the potential for embarrassment and mistrust, the supervisor and the guests appeared to like each other.

## COOPERATIVE FOOD CLUBS

Another formal program utilizing social group work was the Cooperative Food Club. This program was originally conceived out of experience with the emergency food pantry that was responding to the consistent monthly crises and need for food among the very poorest of the wider community. Their resources had not been able to feed them for a full month. In addition, many of them were not taking advantage of food entitlement programs like Food Stamps and WIC. What emerged was a club program which assisted people in becoming connected to entitlement programs, then invited them to become a member of the food club. Members came together in a monthly meeting where they "shopped" for supplementary groceries and where each month there is a presentation on nutrition and budgeting food resources. After two years of the original food club two more clubs were added, La Cooperativa which was conducted in Spanish and The Fugoa, a food club which was an adjunct to a club program for a chronically mentally ill group.

The food clubs were based on the ideas of mutual aid. The highest status in the club seemed to go to those who did the most for the club and other members. For example, the food clubs had a monthly advisory meeting which functioned so that the members had program input, aired grievances, and made suggestions. While it required extra effort to attend those meetings, the most active club members came regularly to care for their club. On the day of the food distribution, jobs were carried out by various members, assigned based on their suitability for such tasks as child care, bagging groceries, setting up, cleaning up, etc. Although those who performed these tasks were rewarded with a small amount of extra food, the bigger reward for them seemed to come out of their service to the club and the status that it brought.

Another way that club members assisted each other was by helping potential members to access food entitlement programs. For example, they might have helped fill out a food stamp application, or taken someone to the WIC office to inquire about eligibility. There was a general appreciation among active club members that membership was extended to those who are doing their best to feed their families by participation in all available programs. Club members appeared proud of that achievement and some were quite eager to share their know-how for program involvement with others.

Club members seemed to share great empathy with one another in the struggle to get by on minimal means. They had no sympathy, however, for "cheaters," and members weeded out suspected abusers with a vengeance.

Groups such as the food clubs need to remain open and flexible. The success of such a program is precariously built on "what works," and when an element is found to be unworkable, it is essential to change it quickly. For example, it was originally required for all club members to participate in the Surplus Commodities distribution program each month. It was soon discovered that the program was often difficult or impossible to enter, so the club dropped that requirement.

The need to constantly evaluate and modify is evidenced by the differences in the three clubs, each of which began as the same basic program, and evolved to meet the needs of the three different groups. The oldest club, the 50 member Originals, had two major sub-groups, older disabled people, most of whom live alone, and young, single-parent families. Most were white. In this club there was extremely high value placed on club service, and they appeared to want to decide on the club rules, the food offered, and educational presentations.

La Cooperativa, a 30 member Spanish speaking club, was made up almost exclusively of Puerto Rican women who were the providers in their families. This group came to get the food, but did not elaborate on the program as the former group did. They enjoyed the relaxation of the thirty minutes while waiting for the food, and were willing to listen to the speakers, but they appeared to be most interested in the food distribution itself, perhaps because their social needs were satisfied in their families and neighborhood.

The Fujoa Club (the group chose the name at its first meeting — it is the misspelled name of a tropical fruit) was run in conjunction with a social program for approximately 12 chronically mentally ill people. While the food distribution was a small motivating factor, it was much more of a social get-together which was perceived as pleasant and safe. Because some members were so fearful, they often needed to be urged to attend. Rather than listening to talks on nutrition, this group usually prepared some food for its own consumption using simple techniques and equipment. With the Fujoa Club, participation in food entitlement programs was treated as an ideal, not a requirement because the group members tended to be scared away and confused by requirements. The club was seen as a warm, caring social hour after which the members went home with groceries and some cooking ideas, but mainly with the assurance that it was a safe place to come back to next month.

Ultimate success in the food clubs seemed to come from no longer needing to participate. In a few cases, people moved to an income level where they were pleased to say they no longer need the program. In all these cases, they expressed gratitude that the food club was there to support their efforts to be good providers when their resources were scarce, and that they were not forced into a demeaning monthly crisis in order to obtain food.

## THE POTENTIAL FOR AIDS PREVENTION

The soup kitchen is a setting in which to test out strategies in self-help with regards to the prevention and early detection of Acquired Immune Deficiency Syndrome (AIDS). The dining room of the soup kitchen is a daily meeting place of many of Middle City's intravenous drug users. They congregate around the coffee pot to talk and drink coffee. A program is now underway to teach a group of guests about the prevention of AIDS, focusing on the issue of the spread of AIDS by the use of contaminated needles and syringes. The self-help program tries to attract the indigenous leaders of the drug-using network so they can talk to their friends about prevention of AIDS through drug rehabilitation, the use of sterile needles for the drug user, and the promotion of sexual practices which are considered safe.

## CONCLUSIONS

In many ways, a soup kitchen is an ideal setting in which to implement social change through the self-help philosophy. Individuals come to the soup kitchen on a regular basis and create an identifiable culture which fosters a sociable, accepting atmosphere. Inevitably, some of the members of the culture become leaders, and some become central figures within social networks.

The concept of both the classes and food clubs does not imply that anyone has a "problem" that needs "treatment." Rather, they embody the spirit of self-help by beginning with the assumption that guests have the ability to share and learn important information and help each other, and the group worker can creatively tap the sharing and helping potential.

The soup kitchen will one day hopefully be an artifact of a just and caring North American society. But until that is so, it can be a place in which to expand and further ideas of self-help with some of the individuals whose lives fall outside of the affluence of the rest of North American society.

## REFERENCES

Bachrach, L.L. "Research Devices for the Homeless Mentally Ill" *Hospital and Community Psychiatry* 35:(9) (September 1984) pp. 910-13.

Behrhorst, Carroll "The Chimaltenango Development Project in Guatemala" in Kenneth Newell (ed.) *Health by the People* W.H.O. 1975 pp. 30-51

Breton, Margot "Reaching and Engaging People: Issues and Practice Principles" *Social Work with Groups* 8(3) (Fall, 1985) pp. 7-21

Britan, Gerald "The Place of Anthropology in Program Evaluation" *Anthropological Quarterly* 51:(1978) 119-128

Cowen, Emory L., Ellis L. Gesten, Mary Boike, Pennie Norton, Alice B. Wilson and Michael A. DeStephano "Hairdressers as Caregivers I" *American Journal of Community Psychology* 7:6 (1979) pp. 633-648

Dumont, M.P. "Tavern Culture: The Sustenance of Homeless Men" *American Journal of Orthopsychiatry* 37 (1967) pp. 938-945

Glasser, Irene *More Than Bread: Ethnography of a Soup Kitchen* Tuscaloosa, Alabama: The University of Alabama Press, 1988

Hartford, Margaret E. *Groups in Social Work* New York: Columbia University Press, 1971

Henderson, J. Neil "Nursing Home Housekeepers: Indigenous Agents of Psychosocial Support" *Human Organization* 40:4 (1981) pp. 300-305

Horn, Joshua S. *Away With All Pests* New York: Modern Reader, 1969

Liebow, Elliot *Tally's Corner: A Study of Negro Streetcorner Men* Boston: Little Brown and Co., 1967

Merry, Sally Engle *Urban Danger: Life in a Neighborhood of Strangers* Philadelphia: Temple Press, 1981

Nanda, Serena *Cultural Anthropology* (second edition) Belmont, California: Wadsworth Publishing Company, 1984

New, Peter Kong-Ming and Yuet-Wah Cheung "The Evolution of Health Care in China: A Backward Look to the Future" *Medical Anthropology* 8:3 (Summer 1984) pp. 169-171

Piven, Frances Fox and Richard A. Cloward *Regulating the Poor* New York: Vintage Books, 1971

Rendle, Gilbert R. Jr. "Welfare, Charity and Ministry: Postures in the Helping Relationship" *The Christian Century* (May 2, 1984) pp. 464-467

Rosenthal, Marilyn M. and Jay R. Greiner "The Barefoot Doctors of China: From Political Creation to Professionalization" *Human Organization* (1982) pp. 330-341

Rousseau, Ann Marie *Shopping Bag Ladies: Homeless Women Speak About Their Lives* New York: Pilgrim Press, 1981

Rubenstein, Carin and Phillip Shaver "The Experience of Loneliness" in *Loneli-*

*ness: A Sourcebook of Current Theory, Research and Therapy* Peplau and Perlman (eds) New York: Wiley, 1982

―――― *The Health of China* Boston: Beacon Press, 1983

Shulman, Lawrence and Alex Gitterman "The Life Model, Mutual Aid, and the Mediating Function in *Mutual Aid Groups and the Life Cycle* Gitterman and Shulman (eds) Itasca, Illinois, F.E. Peacock Publishers, 1986

Sidel, Victor W. and Ruth Sidel *Serve the People* Boston: Beacon Press, 1973

# Empowerment of the Low Income Elderly Through Group Work

## Enid Opal Cox

**SUMMARY.** Older Americans are required to deal directly with multiple changing life circumstances. This paper discusses the nature of powerlessness experienced by many low income older Americans. Isolation and self-blame are frequent outcomes and/or factors in the continuation of this powerlessness. The role of group as the link between isolated elderly and positive interaction with others in their own behalf, and the subsequent lessening of the sense of powerlessness are stressed. Group work in the arenas of income maintenance and survival resources, housing, elder abuse, and health care are suggested as appropriate for the support of elderly struggling to empower themselves vis-à-vis their environment.

Aging in today's America, according to many elderly, "is not for sissies." Most Americans, including older Americans, believe they have little or no power or knowledge to change the environmental situations which affect their lives. Some elderly persons perceive their economic, health, housing, and other problems to be unrelated to those of other people and often due to their own failures or to fate.

Social workers and other community-based practitioners have historically focused their efforts on assisting person-in-environment relationships, and in some cases, on social action aimed at making the environment less hostile to human needs. Group-based interventions are basic to these efforts. In the past two decades, many human service practitioners have witnessed their own feelings of powerless-

Enid Opal Cox, DSW, is affiliated with the Institute of Gerontology, Graduate School of Social Work, University of Denver, University Park Campus, Denver, CO 80208.

ness as this society (a) moves farther away from a commitment to responsibility for the social welfare of its people, (b) dismantles inadequate but critically needed social services, and (c) cuts basic entitlements which are necessary to human survival. Practitioners find themselves in scarce company as they testify at hearings in the attempt to save programs for the poor or middle-income populations. Within this frame of reference, some social work practitioners, psychologists, educators, and researchers, as well as professionals of other helping disciplines, have moved toward interventions which counter this nagging sense of powerlessness. This paper provides an overview of several related theoretical efforts and suggests practice interventions, particularly with groups, which assist elderly clients in their struggle against powerlessness.

Empowerment intervention strategies are defined, for the purpose of this discussion, as those methodological approaches which mobilize consumers of services, their families and communities toward (a) self-care and (b) authentic involvement in the creation of a better environment. The transfer to clients of knowledge and skills necessary for accomplishing these tasks through the use of group work strategies is an essential component of such interventions. In order to focus this discussion on interventions which facilitate empowerment of older people, we will first consider the nature of that powerlessness.

## FACTORS RELATED TO POWERLESSNESS

Powerlessness, or the lack of empowerment among individuals, is based on several factors, according to Sennett and Cobb (1972), and Conway (1979), including: economic insecurity, absence of experience in the political arena, absence of access to information, absence of fiscal support, lack of training in critical and abstract thought, and physical and emotional stress. Learned helplessness, a by-product of our current social service delivery system, is often another contributing factor in developing a sense of powerlessness (Compton and Galaway, 1984). Lerner (1986) develops the concept of surplus powerlessness as "the extent to which one's own emotional, intellectual and spiritual makeup prevents them from actualizing possibilities that do exist." Moreover, Solomon (1976) discusses the role of negative self-image, limited self-knowledge, and negative valuation in the perpetuation of powerlessness.

Feminist literature also provides a wealthy source of material describing the sociological, political, and psychological aspects of powerlessness (Weick and Vandiver, 1982).

The following brief discussion of these contributing factors as they relate to older Americans suggest that many experience a sense of increasing powerlessness in their lives.

### Economic Insecurity and Absence of Fiscal Support

Certainly, statistics report low or diminishing resources for many elderly. While the overall economic picture has brightened considerably for the elderly, large numbers of older persons exist on marginal incomes. In 1984, 12.4 percent of persons aged 65 and older had incomes below the poverty level, and 21.2 percent had incomes below 125 percent of the poverty level. The situation is even worse for selected subgroups of the older population. For example, 46.5 percent of black elderly have incomes below 125 percent of the poverty level (AARP-Senate Committee on Aging, 1986). Insecurity regarding the continuation of the rising cost-of-living related to the fixed or very marginal increases in income of pensions (including Social Security), causes worry for many middle-income elderly. In addition costs of health care including long term nursing home care are the concern of most older Americans.

### Physical and Emotional Stress

Physical and emotional stress are often at high pitch during late life. Physical decline related to aging includes high susceptibility to chronic diseases. "Elderly in the community report a high prevalence of chronic conditions: 44 percent have arthritis, 27 percent have heart conditions, 39 percent have hypertension, 28 percent have a hearing impairment; many have more than one chronic condition" (Rice, 1985). Loss of a spouse and/or other members of one's immediate social support network, poses a tremendous emotional stress for the elderly. Moreover, stress related to role loss involved in retirement, loss of specific family roles, loss of important social positions on boards, committees or in union organizations, etc., presses hard on the value many hold regarding the importance of living "useful" lives.

### Absence of Experience in the Political Arena

While the elderly hold high voting participation records, few have experience in the participatory political activities. Even those more able in the political arena may hesitate to identify with interests of aging constituencies (Atchley, 1985). Access to reliable information concerning policy alternatives is also a great inhibitor to feelings of efficacy. Consequently, many elderly persons believe that they can have no impact through political involvement; they feel, in fact, powerless.

### Insufficient Training in Critical and Abstract Thought

Modern-day socialization and rapid social change has discouraged critical and abstract thought. Accordingly, many elderly have acquired the tendency to rely totally on the opinions of "experts" — health experts, social experts, or financial experts. Many elderly do not seek education regarding health conditions, alternative treatments, and self-care. Additionally, internalized beliefs, attitudes, and preferences concerning appropriate housing or the use of available social and financial resources are often barriers to seeking information or to using services.

### Negative Valuation on Aging

Powerlessness of older Americans is reinforced by the social and psychological pressures attached to the negative valuation in this society placed on aging and being old. Corrigan and Leonard (1978) describe the similar circumstances of elderly in England as follows:

> The social worker must come to terms with the fact that old people experience a structural position which reinforces a useless, wasted feeling. Objectively older people have provided a great deal and should continue to; however, Capitalist society does not recognize this and structurally, old people are locked

into the vicious circle of isolation and uselessness/deterioration/violation.

The complexities of this situation are great. Atchley (1985) notes that "the gerontology literature has consistently shown that older people can accept the stereotypes about aging and the aged and at the same time consider these stereotypes as having no applicability to themselves." For some elderly this ability to separate one's self from the negative valuations of "the elderly" held by society at large helps explain their relatively high self-image. However, it also creates a significant barrier to the organization of older persons around issues related to common needs.

### Role of Social Services: Dependency
### and Learned Helplessness

The nature of social provision in this society, including all aspects of the social service delivery system, has been challenged relative to its role in the creation and maintenance of learned helplessness. Older Americans are well represented among consumers of a social service delivery system wherein programs based on individual means tests tend to be characterized by inadequacies, red tape, stigma, changing eligibility requirements and tenuous fiscal support (Galper, 1975). Dependence on helping systems which are totally out of one's control is often a new and stressful experience for older Americans who have been able to provide for themselves and their families until this point.

The strong belief held by most Americans that people can "make it on their own without government assistance if they really try" tends to reinforce self-blame for economic and/or health crisis. Correspondingly, resources perceived in other societies as rights are regarded as privileges, or, worse, as "hand-outs" in America. A consequence of this continued adherence to rugged individualism rather than group cooperation is that even though our social policy approach to meeting collective needs falls far short of meeting the existing needs, recipients and potential recipients of resources have not organized and are not demanding improved response to their own needs. This lack of group participation in policy decision making increases recipients' sense of alienation, a major component of learned helplessness.

## THEORETICAL BACKGROUND FOR EMPOWERMENT INTERVENTION STRATEGIES

Group oriented empowerment interventions are based on a number of conceptual developments including Schwartz's emphasis on mutual aid (Lee and Swenson, 1986) and the historical evolution of the mainstream model of social work with groups (Papell and Rothman, 1980). Components of this development of special significance to empowerment oriented group work include the emphasis on common goals, mutual aid and non-synthetic experiences. Konopka's (1978) concept of "members" rather than "client" as the appropriate term to describe group membership is also of significance, as is her suggestion of the need for "authenticity, forthrightness, and abrogation of the mystique of professionalism in order to lessen social distance between worker and members." Middleman (1981) demonstrates the critical role of group work strategies in competency-oriented practice through structured groups. The skills groups, theme groups and transition groups she suggests closely resemble the educational and self-help groups suggested in this discussion as appropriate for elderly individuals as a means to empowerment. In addition to these themes related to empowerment Schwartz (1974), in his discussion of private troubles and public issues as a singular focus of social work, reinforces the important principles of empowerment which stress the need for the worker to assume a holistic view of practice. While informed by these basic tenets of group work practice, empowerment oriented practice also gleans important insight from critical/radical social work practice theory, the self-helper and social support movement and work relative to education for critical consciousness (Paulo Friere, 1975).

### Critical/Radical Practice Movement

The critical/radical practice movement in social work is outlined by Galper (1980). Galper identifies the overall goal of social work practice as institutional change, making the important connection between working with individuals and working for social change. Cox and Longres (1981) stress the importance of the "personal as political" as a key element of intervention. Stressing a group orientation, they also note the importance to one's physical and mental health of engaging in an authentic struggle for personal survival and improvement of the quality of one's environment (social change).

The role of the professional social worker in radical/critical practice is viewed as a partnership with the client aimed in the long run toward mutually desirable social change. Expertise here, as in group work, is viewed as being held by both client and practitioner. It is viewed as a resource to be shared. Accordingly, within the critical practice approach to social work with groups, the goal of professionally trained workers is to teach the knowledge and skills which they have acquired to client populations who can in turn be empowered by these skills.

## Self-Help Movement

Gartner and Reisman (1984) suggest several specific findings of the self-help movement which are significant to empowerment interventions. Their observations, based on the "helper therapy" theory, are outlined as follows:

1. The effective helper often feels an increased level of interpersonal competence as a result of making an impact on another's life.
2. The effective helper often feels a sense of equality in giving and taking between himself or herself and others.
3. The effective helper is often the recipient of valuable personalized learning acquired while working with a helpee (frequently concerning a mutual problem).

## Social Support Movement

The social support movement, reflecting the importance of group membership, has also taken active steps in problem areas related to needs of the elderly. According to Johnson and Johnson (1987), and Swenson (1979) social support involves the mutual exchange of resources, such as emotional concern, instrumental aid, information, and feedback. The benefits derived from belonging to a group range from enhanced productivity, psychological well-being and adjustment, and physical health, to the ability to cope with stress, in addition to "the availability of people on whom one can rely for assistance, encouragement, acceptance, and caring." Four examples of support groups appropriate to the elderly population include widow-to-widow programs, care givers support groups, stroke clubs, and arthritis groups. Such group activities have legitimized mutual support or interdependent coping strategies among elderly participants and their families in many areas in which either the client or the family had previously attempted to cope alone.

### Critical Consciousness Education

Many of the intervention strategies used in empowerment approaches are related to the struggle to increase critical consciousness among client constituencies. Critical consciousness refers to people's ability to perceive critically the way they exist in the world with which and in which they find themselves. This includes one's ability to act consciously and critically upon the world—to participate actively in social/environmental change activities. The work of Paulo Friere (1975) on education for critical consciousness represents a significant contribution to empowerment practice.

Corrigan and Leonard (1978) summarize social work implications in regard to increasing critical consciousness among the elderly as follows:

> As with any social work practice, linking individuals with a group or community setting is far from easy, but the collective experience is even more essential for old people. With death and uselessness being experienced in such isolated ways, practitioners must work hard at contradicting this isolation, both in creating group and collective experience and in introducing ideas from the outside (consciousness raising).

## IMPLEMENTATION OF GROUP-ORIENTED EMPOWERMENT PROGRAMS AND STRATEGIES

The perspectives cited above have provided a forceful argument for the development and implementation of empowerment-oriented programs and group interventions in the field of aging. The process of empowerment requires that persons understand their individual struggles in relationship to both their immediate environment (family, housing facility, etc.) and the larger societal context. Group participation is often required to facilitate this comprehension and transformation of personal problems into public issues.

From a holistic perspective, empowerment strategies are needed in a number of specialized arenas for intervention. Figure 1 provides illustrations of a range of interventions relevant to the arenas of income maintenance and survival resources, housing, elder abuse, and health care. These concrete interventions reflect the integration of empowering approaches with group strategies, based on the premise that the problems of powerlessness faced by older Americans cannot be easily addressed in isolation.

The group interventions suggested in Figure 1 that are targeted for poor and/or oppressed elderly have three central characteristics: (a) These groups are self-help task groups or educational groups related to immediate needs/problems of the population, (b) primary targets of group efforts are either external conditions or internalized values which result in feelings of powerlessness, and (c) the activities of these groups address one or more factors of powerlessness noted earlier. The intervention groups suggested by this paper closely resemble education groups or social action groups as described by Toseland and Rivas (1984). Lee (1986) notes relative to her work with homeless women that "people who wanted and needed closer ties, who were frightened of large groups, or who had trouble talking at all needed the service of small groups and groups where something besides talking was the primary vehicle of service." The educational groups most effective with oppressed elderly seek to increase practical knowledge and skills, as well as to develop interpersonal connection and communication skills through group participation. The social action groups most effective for purposes of empowerment include a strong emphasis on self-help which embodies an increasing awareness of common issues and means to remedy environmental stress.

The role of the worker in empowerment group intervention, as in any empowerment strategy, is to achieve the status of "partners" working toward mutually determined goals. This critical status is often not easily achieved. Helper-helpee relationships often rein-

Figure 1

Group Oriented Empowerment Strategies

---

Empowerment Groups in Health Care:

- Organization of social support groups for persons suffering physical disability and for care givers
- Development of educational groups - both patient and professional - for improvements of health related communications
- Development of educational groups focused on Medicare, Medicaid and other potential resources to assist with health care costs

Empowerment Groups in Housing:

- Development of educational groups regarding housing alternatives and home-sharing skills
- Initiation of Crime Watch programs

Empowerment Groups in Elder Abuse:

- Organization of both consciousness raising and social support groups for elders and for their abusers
- Development of self-help groups among care givers

Empowerment Groups in Income Maintenance and other Survival Resources:

- Educational groups focused on Social Security or other income programs
- Organization of cooperatives
- Development of communal gardens
- Encouragement to engage in the struggle for a publicly supported guaranteed base line of resources and employment opportunities

Empowerment Groups Which Develop Intra-Personal Skills:

- Development of group-based skills of conflict resolution and mediation, networking skills, interpersonal skills and organizational skills force feelings of helplessness and dependency. The summary of group activity below provides an example of the evolution of client-worker relationship to the point that both are involved in a mutual struggle to achieve a common goal. In this case, increased low-income housing availability.

Preliminary work undertaken to establish empowerment-oriented groups by the University of Denver's Institute of Gerontology in 1987 indicates that many poor, elderly individuals are initially uncomfortable with group activity. Engagement is often difficult because of negative self-image and/or low levels of trust. In addition, for many of the very old, poor individuals, a life style of taking care of one's self has not included participatory problem-solving processes. In addition to social psychological factors which may inhibit group participation, physical factors, including lack of mobility, pain, hearing impairment, etc., may also pose barriers to participation in group interventions. Consequently, individually focussed empowerment interventions which enhance self-image and competence on an individual level are sometimes prerequisite to interventions involving group activities. Case management assistance may be required for some persons prior to movement toward group-based interactions. Special efforts to provide transportation or to reduce fears associated with disabilities as well as to increase acceptance of disabilities by those group members who are not disabled, are often necessary to successful engagement. The elderly poor have also responded positively to other networking activities such as skills bank or telephone reassurance network membership.

Another critical dimension in regard to empowerment interventions is the level of focus of group activity in regard to a "personal as political" (public/private issue) continuum. For example, in the area of housing, empowerment interventions can focus on any of the following (a) assessment of personal values and feelings that may serve as barriers to the selection of appropriate housing, (b) dealing with an unresponsive landlord, or (c) working with a senior action group to increase the supply of subsidized elderly housing available. The opportunity to overcome powerlessness and related apathy by isolated elderly, even when they are attempting to act in their own behalf, and especially in relationship to complex organizations or political decision making, is often futile without the use of group support. Even the process of validation of one's perspectives is not easy to accomplish alone.

The following example of a group worker's work with elderly individuals in a downtown SRO (Single Room Occupancy hotel) illustrates the need for preliminary work with some elderly poor before linkage to group activities as well as the development of worker-client relationship toward a partnership. The worker, a 30-year-old white male, who was in his second year of an MSW graduate program interviewed all residents willing to participate in the project. Content of the interviews included completion of the Multidimensional Functional Assessment (Duke University, 1978) and segments of appropriate mental health and social support scales. They were also told about the project intent to hold meetings focussed on subjects of interest to the group and to encourage mutual problem-solving. These interviews allowed the worker to gain acquaintance with the individual elderly persons' situations and to begin the establishment of a working relationship.

In one hotel housing 17 elderly residents, a 71-year-old veteran refused to allow the worker into his room. The worker was able, after several contacts, to gain entrance to G's room. G was in critical need of medical care including immediate hospitalization. The worker was able to deal with G's fear of medical care and serve as advocate, visitor and transportation provider throughout G's hospitalization and recovery. Upon his return to the SRO, G joined the group.

Providing linkage to financial or health resources and/or mediation of arguments among residents were common content of such pre-group contacts. One year later, these outreach and helping functions were most often provided by group members other than the leader. Non group members participated through relationships with group members who brought their issues to the group and provided assistance with their problems. Younger residents often sat in on meetings or had their concerns represented by elderly participants. The worker used every opportunity to encourage mutual aid activities among group members.

For all but two of the 13 elderly participants who became regular members of the group, this was their first participation in formal group experiences. Initial meetings were conducted to establish issues of mutual concern to residents. Initially, very little focus was given to problems such as alcoholism, behavioral problems or personal issues such as loss of significant others, etc. Prior assessment of this hotel and others yielded a pattern of isolation, fierce independence and distrust. Consequently, the first group discussions focussed on less threatening common interests such as conditions of the building, or problems with the delivery of meals on wheels (some were left at the front desk and never reached the intended resident). After several weeks, members began to discuss drinking problems related to group attendance. It was low near the first of the month because residents had money to buy alcohol. The worker encouraged checking on absent members to be sure they were not in danger or need of help. As the first year progressed, issues including, for example, lighting, operation of the security systems and the need for recreational activities were addressed by action steps such as the group members requesting an audience with the manager and the owner, trips to local parks, etc. While overt group focus remained on these efforts, the individual group members began to spend more time together outside the group meetings, to attend to each other's personal problems and to exchange material assistance from aspirin to clothing. A recent example involved Ms. A, who was suffering from frightening hallucinations. Two other group members stayed up with her all night. During the first year's activities, the worker's interventions included organization of regular meetings, provision of information about outside resources, encouragement of mutual support and advocacy in individual cases.

In the second year, a more formal educational agenda of information regarding health care, the aging process, political and economic issues, and available resources for the elderly has been introduced. The group is now faced with the very probable demolition of the hotel. The group serves as a focus of information concerning this issue, including the efforts of the Colorado Homeless Coalition and others to save this and other low-income housing units. The group members at this point are expressing a desire to be relocated together if the building cannot be saved. The worker's role is changing from that of expert, advocate and enabler to that of partner with group members as they become involved in the larger mutual issue of low-income housing in the city. While the primary focus has shifted from personal to political aspects of problems the experience in the group also demonstrates that personal and interpersonal issues continue to require simultaneous focus with the political aspects of aging.

## CONCLUSION

Group strategies are essential elements of empowerment interventions. The use of group participation is key to the consciousness raising process. Furthermore, within a group context, work with others in similar circumstances often serves to clarify issues, draw out common problems, identify causes of individual problems and enhance critical exploration of the environment. Groups have the potential for providing the medium through which elderly gain the support necessary for self-acceptance and connection, and in turn, the strength for necessary action. In the process, their perceptions of powerlessness are dispelled and they become mutually empowered.

## REFERENCES

American Association of Retired Persons—U.S. Senate Special Committee on Aging (1985-1986). *Aging America: Trends and projections.*

Atchley, R.O. (1985). *Social forces and aging,* 4th edition. Belmont, CA: Wadsworth.

Compton, B. and Galaway, B. (1984). *Social work processes,* 3rd edition. Homewood, IL: Dorsey Press.

Conway, M. (1979). *Rise gonna rise.* New York: Anchor.

Corrigan, P. and Leonard, O. (1978). Social work practice under capitalism: A Marxist approach. In *Critical texts in social work and the welfare state.* London: MacMillan, Ltd.

Cox, E.O. and Longres, J. (1981). Critical practice—curriculum implications. Council of Social Work Education, Annual Program Meeting, Louisville, KY.

Friere, P. (1975). *Education for critical consciousness.* New York: Seaburn.

Galper, J.H. (1980). *Social work practice: A radical perspective.* Englewood Cliffs, NJ: Prentice-Hall.

Galper, J.H. (1975). *The politics of social service.* Englewood Cliffs, NJ: Prentice-Hall.

Gartner, A. and Reisman, F.E. (Eds.) (1984). *The self-help revolution.* New York: Human Sciences.

Institute of Gerontology (1987). *Interim Report: Elderly Empowerment Project*. Denver: University of Denver Graduate School of Social Work.

Johnson, D.W. and Johnson, F.P. (1987). *Joining together: Group theory and group skills*, 3rd edition. Englewood Cliffs, NJ: Prentice Hall.

Konopka, G. (1978). The significance of social group work base on ethical values. *Social work with groups* 1. 123-131.

Lee, J.A.B. and Swenson, C.R. (1986). The concept of mutual aid. In *Mutual aid groups and the life cycle*. Gitterman, A. and Shulman, L. (Eds.) Itasca, IL: F.E. Peacock. 361-380.

Lee, J.A.B. (1986). No place to go: Homeless women. In *Mutual aid groups and the life cycle*, Gitterman, A. and Shulman, L. (Eds.) Itasca, IL: F.E. Peacock. 245-263.

Lerner, M. (1986). *Surplus powerlessness*. Oakland, CA: The Institute for Labor and Mental Health.

Middleman, R. (1981). The pursuit of competence through structured groups. In *Promoting competence in clients: A new/old approach to social work practice*, Malucio, A. (Ed.) New York: The Free Press.

National Center for Health Statistics. National ambulatory medical care survey. 1981.

Papell, C. and Rothman, B. (1980). Relating the mainstream model of social work with groups to group psychotherapy and the structural group approach. *Social work with groups*. 3(2), 5-23.

Rice, D.P. (1985). Health care needs of the elderly. *Long-term care of the elderly*. Harrington, C., Newcomer, R.J., Estes, C.L. (Eds.). Sage Library of Social Research, *157*. Chap 2. Beverly Hills, CA: Sage.

Schwartz, William (1974). Private troubles and public issues: One social work job or two? In *The practice of social work*, 2nd edition, Klenk, R. and Ryan, R. (Eds.) Belmont, CA: Wadsworth. 82-101.

Sennett, R. and Cobb, J. (1972). *The hidden injuries of class*. Garden City, NY: Vintage.

Solomon, B. (1976). *Black empowerment: Social work in oppressed communities*. New York: Columbia University Press.

Swenson, C.R. (1979). Social networks, mutual aid and the life model of practice. *Social work practice: People and environments*, Germain, C.B. (Ed.) New York: Columbia University Press. 213-238.

Toseland, R. and Rivas, R. (1984). *An introduction to group practice*. New York: MacMillan. 26-37.

Weick, A. and Vandiver, S. (Eds.) (1982). *Women, power and change*. Washington, DC: NASW.

# BOOK REVIEWS

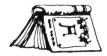

THE PURPOSES OF GROUPS AND ORGANIZATIONS. Alvin Zander. *San Francisco: Jossey-Bass Publishers, 1985, 187 pages.*

This book is another contribution by the author to the knowledge base of practice with groups and a logical development of his life-long work in small group research. He draws upon numerous findings of seemingly disparate concepts investigated by social psychologists, his considerable experience, and observations of groups. He integrates these, demonstrating their influence on the formation of group purposes and the effects of group purpose upon processes, structures and products of group effort. And how needed is a book on group purposes! Group level considerations are minimal in the practice world, to the extent that groups have wandered aimlessly to accomplish some vaguely felt or poorly defined function. New language has been developed which reflects this state of affairs—"focus" groups to distinguish a purposeful group from the prevalent alternative.

The author's intent is to examine purposes of groups and to explain in a systematic, usable fashion their origins and effects. He does this in ten clearly presented, well-structured chapters. Complex ideas are presented simply and concisely without losing the importance of meaning. The book is addressed to scholars, consultants, managers, group leaders, facilitators, trainers.

Zander broadly defines a group as "a collection of individuals who interact with and depend on one another." A group purpose "is that desirable state of affairs that members intend to bring about

through joint efforts." The primary contribution of the book to social workers is application to that group category we label task
groups. This limitation is not claimed by the author, since he includes utility for "psychotherapy" groups among others. Although
many statements of generalization and guidelines presented are directly applicable to such groups, others would need careful exami-
nation when member behaviors, cognitions and affect are the targets for change. This does not suggest that group purpose is not
relevant, but it requires, at least, an analysis of the relationships
between individual values and motives to group purposes. This may
be one area for knowledge development through research, which
the author asks of readers.

After presenting the main ideas of the book, the author explores
the "varied purposes of groups in both ancient times and today, the
reasons for these objectives, and the causes for changes in them."
This chapter is a fascinating historical account which is far-ranging
in examples and different historical eras. For example, information
is presented about societies from 300 B.C. through 1500 A.D. Included are examples from groups in China, early Athens and Rome,
and the early Christian church in Egypt and southern Arabia. In the
second century, societies established by Jewish communities in Eu-
ropean and Middle Eastern nations are analyzed and, later, established trade associations, Vikings and worker guilds are discussed.
The chapter concludes with a review of purposes of groups in current settings. In addition to identifying and describing group purposes historically, the author places the events in their social context. This leads naturally to a separate consideration in Chapter
Three of conditions which foster the formation of groups. Chapter
Four analyzes purposes of groups—their characteristics and how
these differing properties influence member performance. Goal pre-
cision and goal difficulty are two examples provided. Methods by
which a group's purpose is selected are examined in Chapter Five
and the influences of each method upon group performance is suggested. Chapters Six and Seven present the effects of individual
member's values and motives upon group purpose. The process of
evaluating and changing group purposes follows in Chapter Eight.

Of special interest to social workers is Chapter Nine, "Selecting
Group Programs and Activities." The author defines activities as

the group's programs and procedures which are paths to the group's goal. A section on evaluating activities is a contribution to our field. The author provides a way to think about attaining group objectives in relationship to the group's effectiveness and efficiency with attention to the variables of (1) activity objectives, (2) action to achieve those ends and (3) acquisition and use of resources. A set of ratios is presented to analyze activity effectiveness. These ideas are ready for our testing to further practice knowledge. The final chapter is addressed to those who wish to apply the ideas presented in their work with groups.

The day to day practice of social workers includes membership in, consultation to, and/or designation as group leader. We would not tolerate lack of grounding in knowledge about other social units nor should we permit this omission about groups. Thus, this book is a valuable aid in preparation of all social workers. It is particularly important for those assuming positions of administrative leadership in social service delivery systems. Scholars will find hints of a research agenda — the testing of basic assumptions and application of generalizations to social work practice.

*Martha E. Gentry, PhD*
*Associate Professor*
*College of Social Work*
*University of Kentucky, Lexington*

SOCIAL WORK WITH THE AGED AND THEIR FAMILIES. Roberta R. Greene.

"The major objective for this book" writes the author in her preface, "is to develop the social worker's capacity for direct practice with the aged, their families, and the societal agents with whom he/she interacts." To this end, she has organized the book in two sections. Part I deals with a range of informational material designed to give the worker some depth in understanding the problems that may develop for the elderly family member, and to define these problems within the family framework. Part II discusses a range of intervention strategies. These are offered to enable the selection and use of appropriate therapeutic modalities based on a clinical understanding of the behaviors of the individuals involved.

The book is well-written and well-organized. The author has combined several approaches from the various fields of social work and related disciplines to conceptualize a "functional-age model of intergenerational family therapy which provides a holistic and systematic approach to the biopsychosocial problems of the elderly person." She offers an interesting account of the historical and theoretical development of psychosocial casework together with a useful summary of the major contributing concepts in chart form.

A basic and consistent premise of the book is that the elderly person must be viewed within the framework of the family—where there is a family. The author emphasizes the importance of regarding the family system as "the client" and the crisis-connected older member as the "pivotal client rather than the identified patient." Generally speaking, the family of an older person seeks assistance in a time of crisis. Assessment of the crisis, and efforts toward its resolution, must involve recognition of the elderly person's biopsychosocial needs as well as the family's adapting and coping capacities. The worker must view the family as a whole and must understand and empathize with the needs and problems of all its members (e.g., the "sandwich-generation-daughter" torn between the needs of her children, her elderly parent, her husband and herself.) It is necessary to study and understand the background of the problems presented on intake, and to appreciate the family's ongoing and probably long-standing struggle to cope before seeking help. This empathic adaptation of family therapy is both useful and valid.

Also welcome is the author's firm rebuttal of the commonly-held stereotype that modern families do not care for or about their elderly members. Although consistently debunked in gerontological literature, this stereotype seems to prevail in the general community and most certainly affects members of all professions, including social work. Therefore, the true facts cannot be repeated too often.

One of the strengths of this book is its scope. Through her holistic approach, the author recognizes the innumerable facets of her subject, their accompanying interdisciplinary implications and the necessity for social workers to be knowledgeable in all the areas related to a client's functioning. Also identified are the social and societal facets of the current situation, the special needs of special populations (e.g., the old-old, the older woman, problems of the family caring for an Alzheimer's patient, etc.), and some treatment modalities.

A final chapter considers some relevant aspects of supervision. The appendix offers the well-known Palmore quiz on "Facts on Aging," the Kogan "old people scale," and some checklists for supervisors and workers. The bibliography is extensive and identifies some of the better known relevant work in gerontology, family therapy, casework and related fields.

In a sense, the book's strength may also be seen as cause for some inadequacies. It may be said that in its attempt to touch on as many facets of its subject as possible, some ponderous subjects are encapsulated somewhat lightly and even scantily. For example, the question "what is aging?" (which has been the subject of innumerable books and conferences) merits five succinct paragraphs. Social group work, which has become an increasingly important modality in social work, is summarized in a few pages, and only a few possibilities for use cited. The chapter on "Barriers to Service Delivery" speaks of ageism, social attitudes, myths and stereotypes, countertransference and death anxiety—but fails to identify the larger picture of a fragmented social system whose priorities do not seem to focus on human needs. In these, as in other chapters, the author has summarized some important practice and research, but has not indicated to the reader how much more there is to be learned about these truly significant dimensions of her subject. It would have given her book even greater magnitude had she in some way acknowledged this. Also, the book is somewhat sparsely illustrated with case examples which link living practice to theory and translate abstractions into realities. The book would be enhanced by more of these.

Despite some such few limitations, this volume is welcomed as one which provides an overview and a fine human approach to a very important subject. Broadly conceived, it combines some significant research from a number of relevant areas and presents a well-integrated approach to understanding and helping elderly clients and their families.

From this reviewer's viewpoint and experience, these concepts are not as "new" or different as the author suggests. Many practitioners in the field of aging have, for some time, adapted, borrowed and synthesized approaches and have utilized methods from family therapy, systems theory, community organization, and group work among others. It is useful, however, to find these identified and recorded in a single volume such as this and the whole becomes greater than the sum of its parts.

This book is recommended as a useful text for graduate students in social work and other helping disciplines such as nursing, counseling, psychology and medicine among others.

*Shura Saul, EdD, ACSW*

THE SELF-HELP SOURCEBOOK: FINDING AND FORMING MUTUAL AID SELF-HELP GROUPS. Edward J. Madara and Abigail Meese, Editors and Compilers. *Denville, NJ: St. Clares-Riverside Medical Center, 1986, 140 pages, paper.*

This book is a current and fairly comprehensive resource of self-help groups and organizations. The editors expand a directory of self-help groups in New Jersey (which was originally compiled in 1979) into a national directory. All but twenty pages of this sourcebook includes this resource directory. This compilation consists of a list of self-help clearinghouses throughout the United States; a list of specific self-help resources (over 400) categorized under addictions/dependencies, bereavement/death, health/disabilities, mental health, parenting/family, and others; a separate list of resources for rare disorders; a list of toll-free helpline resources; and a nineteen-page index for easy reference to all of the resources described. The group category listings provide information particularly useful for finding an appropriate self-help group. Each item summarizes the purpose of the group or organization, the services it offers, the data for contacting the resource, the date it was organized, the number of nationwide or worldwide chapters, and the date on which this information was obtained and verified. For example, under the *Parenting/Family* category, one finds the following:

> TOUGH LOVE* Self-help program for parents, kids, and communities, for dealing with the out-of-control behavior of a family member. Parent support groups help parents take a firm stand with their kids. Quarterly newsletter $10/year. Guidelines for starting groups. Write: Tough Love, Box 1069, Doylestown, PA 18901. Call (215) 348-7090. Organized 1980. 1500 groups internationally. 10/85.

Additionally, this book includes an introduction by Phyllis Silverman designed to define self-help groups and a brief section by Edward J. Madara entitled "How-to Ideas for Developing Groups." In her introduction, Silverman suggests that "mutual help" is a more appropriate term for groups in which people who share a problem or predicament come together to help one another through support and information. Madara's section focuses on how individuals can start such mutual help groups and on how professionals can function as consultants in developing these.

As far as it goes, this book is a useful resource for individuals seeking a self-help resource or for professional referral purposes. I wish, however, the book had gone further than this objective, as implied in the "sourcebook" title.

The editors offer little to explain and clarify the nature of these significant resources. The sheer volume of the lists reflects that self-help resources have grown geometrically over the last two decades. Why? Silverman hypothesizes that this movement evolves from a need to "humanize" and "democratize" services partly in reaction to bureaucratic professionalism's tendency to depersonalize consumers. Indeed, what distinguishes the groups and organizations listed in this directory are the criteria for their inclusion: they are composed of "peers," people who share a common experience or situation; they are primarily run by and for its members, who have a sense of "ownership" for the group or network being theirs; and they are voluntary and non-profit (they charge dues or raise money but do not charge fees for services).

Alcoholics Anonymous (A.A.) — the prototype of self-help groups and organizations — began in 1935 to provide mutual support through sharing experiences, strengths, and hopes for members to solve common problems and help each other recover from alcoholism. Today, A.A. has 32,000 groups in the United States and 63,000 groups worldwide. The A.A. story and this book suggest that the self-help group model is a powerful resource, especially attractive to persons undergoing stressful transitions in particular social roles — patients with particular diseases, recovering alcoholics, former mental patients, or new parents. This directory of over 400 such self-help groups attests to the increased intensity needs for empowering, mutual aid relationships in conjunction with practical help in contemporary society. Those of us who study the small group as a resource in professional practice can learn much from these current trends in self-help groups. Those of us facing very practical crisis in our own social roles can be heartened at the possibility of finding or forming such a self-help group among the resources potentially useful to our successful coping with such problems in living. We will likely find this book very useful in both respects, although we can expect more questions than answers when we read this from the scholar rather than consumer perspective.

The editors imply that these criteria enhance the possibility of these self-help groups as mutual aid resources for members. Yet, they offer no evidence for this hypothesis. If mutual aid is the central dynamic for help in these groups, as the editors suggest, it is difficult to fathom how groups established primarily for public educational purposes (e.g., Nat'l. Assoc. for Sickle Cell Disease, Inc.), those designed for advocacy (e.g., Stop Abuse By Counselors), and those which offer phone support, newsletters, and a pen pal network (e.g., Concerned United Birthparents) are comparable to those which develop interactional self-help groups (e.g., National Black Women's Health Project/Self-Help Division).

In sum, this book serves well the function for "finding" self-help resources, as suggested in the subtitle, but seems especially inadequate in the theory base for "forming" such groups. It is thus much more of a directory than a sourcebook.

*Joseph D. Anderson, DSW*
*Professor*
*Shippensburg University*
*Senior Teaching Fellow, National University of Singapore*

RECREATIONAL LEADERSHIP: GROUP DYNAMICS AND INTERPERSONAL BEHAVIOR. 2nd Edition. Jay S. Shivers. *Princeton: Princeton Book Company, 1986, 416 pages, hard cover.*

"Leadership," I remember learning from Cartwright and Zander's text on group dynamics, "is the performance of those acts that help a group to accomplish its goals." At the time, I found this particular view of leadership to be a satisfactory definition for a social group worker. We were always striving to teach, model and support leadership behaviors performed by group members, in the belief that the best group worker was the one who led the least; the one who successfully engaged members in taking responsibility for the management of their own group through participation in a shared process of democratic leadership. Now Shivers has brought together a broad-ranging discussion of this fascinating and complex subject, that goes far beyond the Cartwright and Zander definition. In his book, he provides a thorough-going up-to-date review of relevant social science research and theory as it relates to recreational practice. His purpose, he writes, is to:

> . . . explain the characteristics of the leader, to describe the situations which call him into being, and to define leadership and its essential components for practical use and study . . .

and to "translate" this research and theory into "correct practice" for leaders in the field of recreation.

The book is organized into four major sections, so as to deal, in turn, with leadership and the individual, the group, the organization, and the general subject of effectiveness as a leader. He begins with a discussion of leadership in recreation, a field that has the goal of "helping people achieve happiness, an optimistic view of life, and relief from stress." Noting that confusion exists between influence and leadership, Shivers opts for a democratic approach, rather than one in which people are led by threat or intimidation. He then discusses theory and research on leadership, including the work on the traits that supposedly make for leadership, the idea that the leader is a "central figure" within a group, studies on different kinds of situations that require different styles of leadership, and the view of leadership as a set of functions that can be carried out by any member of a group. The body of knowledge reported on in this chapter becomes the book's touchstone, and is referenced and elaborated upon thereafter.

In order to examine leadership in the fullest sense, Shivers first relates his topic to individual factors that affect communication, such as empathic ability, awareness of the social veneer others use to protect themselves, and the place of testing in relationship development. He also discusses the ways in which one individual influences another through domination, power and/or influence. Here he is particularly interested in the ways in which individuals come to voluntarily change attitudes and behaviors.

In his discussion of leadership and the group, the author describes different ways that individuals become recognized as group leaders, and takes the position that group action requires a leader — someone who can speak for the group — and that most groups recognize and accept this fact. Leadership is then discussed in relation to a number of group dynamics, including the relationship between the individual and the group, group cohesiveness, and the group as reference point for its members. He discusses the many roles played by a leader, and how these roles interact with the kind of group being led, i.e., task group, social-action group, problem-solving group, and client-centered group. At this point, his discussion of the leadership techniques that could be used in such groups uses a broad-brush approach, and lacks the kind of specific guidelines that could instruct the reader in the "correct practice" of leadership.

In discussing leadership in organizations, he says that the trait theory of leadership, once esteemed, then subsequently de-valued as too simplistic, may have some value after all. In fact, current research suggests, he says, that there is an interplay between the group's makeup, the social situation in which the group exists, the group's task, *and* the attributes of the leader. He then proceeds to describe the desirable attributes of leaders who run recreational organizations, including such things as the desire to be a leader, intelligence (including verbal skill, sensitivity to others, the ability to discern right from wrong, empathic ability, and so forth), good appearance, good mental health, and a number of "good" character traits (such as loyalty, integrity, discretion, and so forth). No doubt the attributes of a leader do interact with other factors to influence that leader's effectiveness, but one does not have to be a paragon to lead. The trouble with the trait theories was that they oversimplified a complex issue. Shivers says he knows this, yet proceeds to postulate certain basic attributes of recreational leaders, once again oversimplifying the issue. In the rest of this section, Shivers describes leadership at different levels of the organization, including the functional (line-worker), supervisory and managerial levels.

The final section of the book deals with leadership effectiveness. He begins with a discussion of challenges faced by leaders, e.g., hidden enemies, polarized factions, and so forth, and errors that leaders typically make, e.g., compromising principles for immediate gain, behaving in an arrogant manner, indecisiveness and so forth. He describes the "underlying activities every leader must undertake," as (1) challenging the accepted, (2) having an inquiring mind, (3) showing a common touch, (4) creating a feeling of unity, and (5) promoting cohesiveness. What follows is an elaboration of these points which, for the reader, says — these are the many things you have to think about and be aware of it you want to be an effective leader. The book concludes with a discussion of the ways in which leadership can be evaluated.

Those who practice social work with groups, who administer such programs, or who teach about such endeavors would do well to add this book to their collection. Shivers has done an effective job of reviewing the whole subject of leadership in a comprehensive and thoughtful way. In a classroom, for example, any of his chapters could provide the basis for a thoroughgoing discussion of leadership issues. What the book does not provide as well are clear guidelines for how to "practice correctly," in the sense of being able to size up a situation, and respond to it in a way that will move a group or organization along toward the achievement of its goals. Scattered throughout the book are a number of examples in which recreationists deal with situations requiring effective leadership, but these often amplify a conceptual point, rather than providing a model for the translation of theory into practice. On balance though, the book provides an excellent discussion of leadership, with implications for all professionals who find themselves struggling with the demands of leading others effectively.

*Harvey Bertcher, DSW*
*Professor of Social Work*
*University of Michigan School of Social Work*